YOU WERE NOT
BORN TO SUFFER

ALSO BY BLAKE D. BAUER

Intentions In Gratitude

YOU WERE NOT BORN TO SUFFER

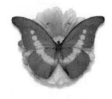

Love Yourself Back To Inner Peace,
Health, Happiness & Fulfillment

Blake D. Bauer

BALBOA.
PRESS

A DIVISION OF HAY HOUSE

Balboa Press books may be ordered through booksellers or by contacting:

Balboa Press
A Division of Hay House
1663 Liberty Drive
Bloomington, IN 47403
www.balboapress.com
1-(877) 407-4847

Because of the dynamic nature of the Internet, any web addresses or links contained in this book may have changed since publication and may no longer be valid. The views expressed in this work are solely those of the author and do not necessarily reflect the views of the publisher, and the publisher hereby disclaims any responsibility for them.

The author of this book does not dispense medical advice or prescribe the use of any technique as a form of treatment for physical, emotional, or medical problems without the advice of a physician, either directly or indirectly. The intent of the author is only to offer information of a general nature to help you in your quest for emotional and spiritual well-being. In the event you use any of the information in this book for yourself, which is your constitutional right, the author and the publisher assume no responsibility for your actions.

Any people depicted in stock imagery provided by Thinkstock are models, and such images are being used for illustrative purposes only.
Certain stock imagery © Thinkstock.

Printed in the United States of America

ISBN: 978-1-4525-6259-9 (sc)
ISBN: 978-1-4525-6261-2 (hc)
ISBN: 978-1-4525-6260-5 (e)

Library of Congress Control Number: 2012921142

Balboa Press rev. date: 10/17/2013

Beyond the beliefs of any religion,
There is the truth of the human spirit.
Beyond the power of nations,
There is the power of the human heart.
Beyond the ordinary mind,
The power of wisdom, love, and healing energy is at work in the universe.
When we can find peace within our hearts,
We contact these universal powers.
This is our only hope.

—TARTHANG TULKU, TIBETAN BUDDHIST LAMA

To you, the reader.

May you be at peace in your heart, healthy, happy, fulfilled, and free.

And also to our world, which is crying out for our love and compassion.

May we all learn to love ourselves, each other, and all life unconditionally.

TABLE OF CONTENTS

There are two basic motivating forces: fear and love. When we are afraid, we pull back from life. When we are in love, we open to all that life has to offer with passion, excitement, and acceptance. We need to learn to love ourselves first, in all our glory and our imperfections. If we cannot love ourselves, we cannot fully open to our ability to love others or our potential to create. Evolution and all hopes for a better world rest in the fearlessness and openhearted vision of people who embrace life.

—JOHN LENNON

WELCOME

At what point do we finally declare that we have suffered enough? When do we finally proclaim enough misery, enough sickness, and enough settling for less than we are worthy, deserving, and capable of?

Must we face a life-threatening illness, financial ruin, the destruction of our relationships, or the deep depression, anxiety, and insecurity that result from living in denial or fear? Must we constantly numb ourselves with alcohol, antidepressants, drugs, food, and material possessions?

What is it that defines the moment when a person wholeheartedly asserts that he or she deserves the best in life and thus will not accept anything less? When is enough truly enough? And if not now, then when?

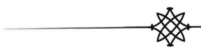

As I am sure you can relate, I saw a great deal of suffering as a child. In fact, I watched many of my own family members unintentionally destroy themselves, their lives, and their loved ones. I saw a lot of sadness, anger, and pain in the eyes of those around me. I saw people who didn't smile nearly as much as they would cry. I saw people who weren't happy or satisfied with their jobs, their relationships, or the lives they had created.

As a young man I had no idea I was just like all of these people. I didn't know I was already heading down the same self-destructive path they were on. Instinctually, what I did know was that I wanted something different. Deep in my heart I somehow knew it was possible to create a fulfilling life that I loved even if no one was going to show me how to make it happen.

For most of us growing up, our role models do not embody the peace, health, or happiness that we all, deep down, know to be our destiny and our birthright. Rather, we witness a significant amount of misery, disharmony, and unhealthy compromise. Both literally and metaphorically, we look up to people who settle for less than they are worthy, deserving, and capable of.

Personally, in my own heart, I knew I did not want to end up like that. I don't believe any of us do. Deep down, I believe we all come into this world *knowing that we were not born to suffer.* I believe that in our heart of hearts we all know that life is meant to be lived and enjoyed with purpose, awareness, respect, and love.

Fortunately, we live during a time in human evolution when more and more of us are reconnecting to this inner knowing that we temporarily lost touch with. All across the globe, humanity is remembering extremely empowering inner truths that we've been ignoring for way too long.

We're remembering that we were born to love life and to live our lives to the fullest, with love for ourselves, love for other people, and love for our world, because life was meant to be a deeply wonderful and beautiful experience, not one that is defined by fear, misery, isolation, sickness, poverty, and war.

Life undoubtedly brings with it struggles, but it's how we choose to address these challenges that ultimately determines the quality of our daily lives. How we approach our psychological, emotional, and physical pain, therefore, either leads us toward inner peace, health, happiness, and fulfillment or into depression, anxiety, anger, and regret.

Thus, each day we are given a choice.

Do we remember that we did not come here to suffer? Do we remember that we deserve the best in our relationships, our careers, and our health, and that we have everything we need within us to claim this? Do we remember that we deserve to be treated with kindness, love, and respect both by ourselves and by others?

Or, do we settle for a half-lived life? Do we compromise ourselves and abandon our soul's inner calling? Do we betray our inner truths and constantly allow other people to dishonor, take advantage of, and disrespect us?

Looking at this choice objectively, it doesn't seem like much of a choice at all. I would wager my life that every person who reads this would choose the first option and honor it all the time if they knew that everything would work out along the way.

Unfortunately, however, most of us do not value ourselves deeply enough yet to claim the high quality of life that's waiting for every single one of us. We haven't cultivated a strong enough faith and trust in ourselves, in life, in the universe, or in God to wholeheartedly go after what we want and love in life.

As a result, most of us just settle for less than we're worthy, deserving, and capable of, and then we suffer for it.

But life doesn't have to be this way.

Believe nothing. No matter where you read it, or who said it, even if I have said it, unless it agrees with your own reason and your own common sense.

—BUDDHA

MY INSPIRATION

You Were Not Born to Suffer was born out of my personal quest for two things in life. The first was liberation from my own psychological, emotional, and physical suffering. The second was my unquenchable desire for the truth—the truth about life, the truth about myself, and most importantly, the truth about my life's destined purpose.

Who am I? Why am I here? What is the purpose of life, and of my life in particular? How do I heal myself and find freedom mentally, emotionally, physically, financially, and spiritually?

How and where can I find lasting inner peace, vital health, happiness, fulfillment, and true love? How can I thrive every day rather than just get by and survive? How can I create a joyful, successful, and prosperous life without settling for anything less?

After over a decade of answering these questions, while professionally supporting thousands of people internationally to do the same, the empowering insights I've discovered form the foundation for the pages that follow.

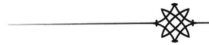

I was not completely aware of it at the time, but as a young man I suffered quite deeply within myself, mostly psychologically and emotionally, but also physically at times. My early life, like many of our lives, had presented its fair share of painful experiences and confusing situations.

On top of the challenging experiences I encountered as a growing child, I created a significant amount of pain for myself as a teenager in my attempts to run from, deny, and numb myself both to the pain within me and also to the painful situations around me. By the time I was eighteen years old I had set in motion a domino effect that had caused my world to crumble. I had been suspended from high school on three different occasions. I had been arrested for drug possession three different times. I was also asked to resign as a captain of my high school football team three games into my senior season after being arrested for driving under the influence of alcohol.

Around this same time, I was also unfaithful to my high school girlfriend while largely under the influence of pharmaceutical drugs for which I did not have a prescription or a valid need for taking. Even though I loved and cared for her very deeply, I unintentionally broke her heart through my unconscious and self-destructive behavior.

As a teenager, I was completely out of control. I created a significant amount of pain not only for myself but also for those people closest to me. I had no idea that I was running from myself, my life, and my painful past. I didn't know I was denying, avoiding, and numbing myself to the psychological and emotional pain that lived within me which I had never healed from my childhood and earlier teenage years.

Consequently, just before graduating from high school, I had broken my own heart wide open and lost the two most important aspects of my lived reality: I lost the girl I loved, and I also lost the game of football I loved. At this point in my development, these two aspects of my life comprised the majority of my identity, or my ego, and within a very short period I had unintentionally pushed them both away. In retrospect I came to see that through these events I had lost my sense of self, or who I thought I was. I didn't know this then, but I had experienced what is most often referred to in psychological and spiritual thought as a "death of self," where the idea or the image of who we think and believe ourselves to be is completely shattered.

Reflecting back on it now, as hard as this time in my life was, I'm so grateful for what I experienced, because it set in motion the birth of my true self as well as the discovery of my life's destined purpose. Without the pain I had experienced as a child and the further pain that I created as a teenager, I would not be in a place today where I'm able look back on this part of my life with a deep understanding of the purpose it served in the unfolding of my destiny.

I now know that I had to lose myself in order to heal myself and truly find myself.

Moving forward after high school, I left home for college still carrying with me my largely unconscious psychological and emotional pain. I went away to college because it was expected of me both by my family and also by my local community.

The larger majority of the people graduating from the high school I attended were going on to college. I had no real idea of who I was or what I wanted to do with my life. I just unconsciously went with the flow.

I began taking business and advertising classes, thinking I wanted to make a lot of money, as money seemed to be a very important aspect of life, if not the most. My family and the community I was raised in valued money and making money greatly, and I had developed an unconscious drive to live up to excessively high financial standards and expectations.

As so many of us do, I unconsciously believed that money alone equaled both success in life as well as freedom. And so my initial intentions during my first year of college were driven by a desire for financial wealth above all else.

It wasn't too long, however, before I realized that my motives were ultimately empty and meaningless, and that underneath my "normal" outer life circumstances, I was extremely lost and suffering quite deeply within myself.

After my second year of studies I finally found the courage to leave college, step into the unknown, and follow what became an unquenchable desire to heal myself on all levels of my being.

Intuitively I knew in my heart that life wasn't meant to be as empty or painful as I was experiencing it to be. I just knew without doubt that there was a way out of my suffering and confusion into a clear and joyful state of being.

At the same time I also held a deep knowing that my life had a meaningful purpose and that I would find it if only I searched long and hard enough for it. Somehow I just knew that I could create a passionate and fulfilling life for myself where I was truly at peace, healthy, and happy each and every day.

And so my quest began.

My search for truth, healing, and clarity of purpose led me to a number of alternative universities and learning institutions. I also continued my studies privately with various spiritual teachers, psychotherapists, traditional shamans, herbalists, and energetic healers. I formally studied at two different schools for acupuncture and Oriental medicine while simultaneously working with and for a group of Chinese medical doctors. I also visited a number of physicians, alternative healers, and therapists to help me understand, transform, and heal things in myself that I struggled to understand, transform, and heal on my own. I attended a variety of trainings, lectures, workshops, and retreats that focused on alternative healing techniques and spiritual disciplines. I intensively studied and practiced various forms of meditation, qi gong, yoga, and tai chi on a daily basis for years.

I became so passionately hungry to understand myself and my life. I read book after book on spirituality, religion, God, philosophy, psychology, biology, physics, enlightenment, the evolution of consciousness, nutrition, alternative medicine, and various forms of energetic healing. All I wanted was to free myself from my psychological, emotional, and physical suffering and find a clear purpose in my life.

Throughout these years following my decision to leave behind a "conventional" career and life path, I began to retreat more and more from the outer world and travel deeper into the depths of my own being—into my body, my mind, my heart, and my soul. Like a wounded animal in deep need of healing, I isolated myself from friends and family. Organically, I came to live like a monk and focused for hours each day practicing the various self-awareness and self-healing practices that I had studied and learned. My search for truth, freedom, and clarity of purpose became the focus of all my time and energy.

After roughly six years of concentrating solely on these pursuits I had gratefully reached a certain level of clarity, peace, and joy within myself. Through studying the various healing modalities and spiritual practices that I had so intensively, I learned a great deal about healing myself and consciously creating a healthy, happy, and fulfilling life.

Eventually I came to see that everything I had learned in my own quest for well-being, purpose, and freedom directly transferred over and gave me deep insights into how I could support and guide others in their own healing processes, as well as in their own search for true meaning and purpose in life. I found that as I discovered deeper levels of peace, health, joy, clarity, and passion within myself I naturally became inspired to support others to find and create the same for themselves. In fact, I realized that nothing moved me more than connecting with another human being openheartedly and honestly with a genuine intention to help.

As time progressed, I found more and more purpose in sharing what I had learned with others to help them heal and transform their own lives in positive and fulfilling ways. I came to feel that there was really nothing more important in life than being at peace, healthy, happy, fulfilled, purpose driven, loved, and loving, and so I felt both inspired and also responsible to share with other people what I had been blessed to discover within and for myself.

By this point in my journey I felt that I had, for the most part, found my life's purpose in supporting other people to heal themselves, discover their own life purpose, and find inner freedom. However, at the core of my being, I still was not as clear or as motivated within myself each day as I wanted to be; I could feel there was still more to my unfolding destiny that I was not aware of.

In my heart I was certain that one day I would clearly discover my purpose for living—the true reason why I was born and the reason why I was on this planet. At this stage I knew I had not totally grasped what this was yet, but I also knew that one day soon I would indeed find the one thing I was born to wake up every morning for and focus all of my energy on without doubt and without any form of external direction whatsoever.

I am very grateful to say that the book you now hold in your hands represents me finally finding what I was looking for.

Toward the end of 2008 I was transitioning into sharing with and teaching others what I had discovered and learned on a full-time basis. I was living in Boulder, Colorado, USA, and I had just begun building a private practice with the intention of supporting others to heal themselves and consciously transform their lives.

Around this same time, through a number of very synchronistic events, I unexpectedly decided to attend a training seminar in Australia on a unique form of energetic medicine and kinesiology being taught by a wonderful doctor, healer, and teacher. Even though I had never been interested in traveling to Australia for any reason, out of nowhere, I felt so strongly about flying across the world to be at this training. I was interested in the seminar and of course in the man who was teaching it, but I strangely and deeply felt that the training was not the main reason why I was destined to attend. At times I had felt that I might meet my soul mate, but I wasn't certain of anything besides the fact that I needed to go; at least that much was clear to me.

This unforeseen trip across the world ended up being life changing in so many ways. Reality-shattering and heart-opening experiences unfolded in front of me one after another. In fact, the most significant of these experiences became a primary catalyst for this book. I did indeed meet a beautiful woman at the training named Maxine, who turned out to be a soul mate with whom I've shared many past lives. Without going into too much detail, Maxine became my life partner and my best friend relatively quickly. What is vitally necessary to express here is that meeting Maxine opened my heart to love in a way words will never do justice in expressing. She was the key that unlocked both my heart and my destiny.

My experiences of loving Maxine and being loved by Maxine reflected back to me the infinite source of unconditional love within me that I came to realize was my soul's deepest nature. On the second evening that Maxine and I spent time together I heard the words, *"Once I love myself unconditionally, loving another becomes an act of self-love."* One might say that these words "came through" me, or that the voice of God and the universe expressed them from within me. Regardless of how we choose to look at it, at this point I didn't fully comprehend how profound these words truly were. But without hesitation I grabbed a pen and wrote them down, because I could instinctually feel the power and significance contained within them.

A few days later, on my flight back to the United States from Australia, I opened the journal in which I had written, *"Once I love myself unconditionally, loving another becomes an act of self-love,"* and I proceeded to write what became the seed for this book.

I had not yet realized that a large part of my ultimate purpose in life was to write a book that illuminated how loving ourselves unconditionally in every moment, situation, and relationship is the most direct path to our psychological, emotional, physical, financial, and spiritual freedom and then teach its empowering message. I just began writing.

Back in Boulder, Colorado, however, not too long after my return from Australia, it became crystal clear to me that I was destined to write a book that focused on cultivating unconditional love, kindness, and compassion for ourselves as the path to healing ourselves, fulfilling our life purpose, and realizing our greatest potential. Having searched so intensively for this deep inner knowing and for the resulting clarity and freedom that I was certain were possible, when it finally surfaced, I just knew in my heart, without any doubt, that writing this book and sharing this message was what I came here to do.

The insights I began having into loving oneself unconditionally as the key to everything that we seek in life seemed to be the last piece to this puzzle I had been putting together for years. I could see that in my own restless quest for truth, healing, and clarity of purpose I had merely been learning to love myself unconditionally. It became so clear that sharing what I had learned in the format of a book would be the most effective way to inspire, empower, and support as many people as possible globally to love, help, and heal themselves.

Up until this particular point in my life I had often felt like I was stuck in a big, confusing maze, one that I was always struggling to find a way out of. I knew there was an exit out of the frustration and confusion that represented life in this "maze," but no matter where I went or what I did I could never find complete and lasting freedom.

What became crystal clear to me when I finally found the answer I had been seeking for years was that it had been within me and present all along. As most of us do, I had believed that this "thing" I was searching for was outside of myself somewhere in the outer world, when in reality it was always within me, just waiting to be discovered and brought forth fully into my life.

Thankfully, I finally grasped the fact that the only way out of this confusing "maze" that we call life was to go even deeper into myself. Although I had heard it before, this was the point where I wholeheartedly realized that *the only way out is the way in.*

Like a bird that continually flies into a glass window and hurts itself because it doesn't see the window, I had created a tremendous amount of pain and disappointment for myself because I kept looking externally for something that could only be found in the depths of my own heart and soul. Thank God, I finally realized that no lasting peace, happiness, fulfillment, or freedom could be found in other people or other places—and definitely not in the "things" of the world.

Following these realizations I continued to have intense and beautiful experiences of love in my relationship with Maxine that not only showed me the powerful healing potential of love, but which constantly confirmed to me that my soul's true nature actually is love—that I am, *as we all are,* an abundant source of pure, unconditional love.

Like all of us unconsciously do, I also realized that I had lived my whole life like a puppy dog chasing its tail. *I was ultimately just looking for love, when in fact I was love itself.* In awakening to this universal and fundamental truth, I realized that the path to finding the abundant source of love within us, which is also the path to embodying the love that we are, is one that requires all of us to answer the evolutionary call to master loving ourselves unconditionally.

With this awareness dominating my consciousness, I continued my exploration into what it truly means to love myself, and to love oneself, unconditionally. After each empowering realization came a crucial period of deep healing and integration, where I learned to embody the self-awareness necessary to live and act in the world with unconditional self-love. Through relating to myself in this compassionate way, I found the most profound levels of healing, joy, and inner freedom that I've ever experienced. And that is why I chose to write this book: to share with you what I've discovered to be the most valuable key to consciously creating a healthy, happy, and fulfilling life that is full of passion, purpose, and love.

Throughout the following pages I will share with you everything I have learned about unconditional self-love from both my own healing and spiritual journey as well as from my professional success with thousands of people internationally to date. The practical insights offered throughout this book are intended to support you in breaking through any and all fears you might have so you can finally liberate yourself from your psychological, emotional, and physical suffering and come to enjoy this gift that we call life.

I'd like to thank you for reading *You Were Not Born to Suffer,* because as you master loving yourself unconditionally you will indeed find the abundant source of peace, health, happiness, and fulfillment within the depths of your being. As you do so, you will bring this inner wealth with you everywhere you go, making our world a much better place for everyone. And for this, I am eternally grateful.

With all my heart, I hope you enjoy.
Blake D. Bauer
Newtown, Victoria, Australia
October 2012

You can search throughout the entire universe for someone who is more deserving of your love and affection than you are yourself, and that person is not to be found anywhere. You, yourself, as much as anybody in the entire universe, deserve your love and affection.

—BUDDHA

WHAT DO YOU THINK ABOUT SELF-LOVE?

As I'm sure you've already realized for yourself, most of us never learned how to relate to ourselves with unconditional love, kindness, and compassion. The majority of us don't even know that it's possible to love ourselves in healthy and conscious ways, let alone what doing so daily would actually entail.

Quite simply, very few of us ever had people in our lives growing up that embodied a healthy example of what it means to live and act in the world from a place of unconditional self-love. In fact, for generations all across the globe, self-love has been judged and shunned as a negative and selfish way of being in the world, primarily because very few people actually understand what it means to love oneself unconditionally or why it is so important to master.

We can't blame anyone for self-love's negative reputation, because no one knows any better. If anyone did, they would (1) love themselves unconditionally and (2) always encourage others to do the same.

The ultimate truth underneath our common collective judgments and resistance to loving ourselves unconditionally, or to allowing others to love themselves unconditionally, is that we're all merely protecting ourselves from feeling emotional pain. More specifically, we all subconsciously fear what we do not love within ourselves, our lives, and our past, because we fear feeling the emotional pain that we ourselves have created by relating to ourselves so aggressively, critically, and self-destructively throughout our lives.

In other words, the unconscious relationship that the majority of us have with and toward ourselves is really the one dynamic that keeps us at war inside ourselves, constantly feeling hurt, angry, powerless, anxious, guilty, ashamed, stressed, unhappy, unhealthy, and unsatisfied because we know that in the past we have not related to ourselves with the unconditional love, kindness, and compassion that we both desire and deserve.

Personally, I believe we'll all eventually realize that viewing self-love as negative or selfish is one of the most detrimental perspectives that exists within human consciousness. If we do not have a relationship with ourselves that is based on unconditional love, kindness, and compassion, it's not only impossible for us to feel good and enjoy our lives, it's also impossible for us to relate to other people from a place of unconditional love, kindness, and compassion as well.

It is crucial for all of us to understand that our inner relationship with ourselves ultimately determines how we relate to everyone and everything in the world around us. If our relationship with ourselves is unconscious, unhealthy, or destructive, then our relationships to other people and to all life will undoubtedly be unconscious, unhealthy, and destructive as well.

The liberating truth that both heals us and unites us globally is that every single person alive struggles to love themselves fully and unconditionally. You, me, the men and women around you right now, wherever you are—your family members, your friends, your neighbors, your colleagues, your boss, your employees, your children, and definitely your parents, even your parents' parents, and their parents too, all struggle, or have struggled, to relate to themselves from a place of unconditional self-love.

It's just the way it is.

Or rather, it's the way it has been. I say this because collectively the whole human family is waking up now. We're not only ready for it; we're ravenously hungry for a new way of life. Deep down, we're all ready for new ways of relating to ourselves, to each other, and to our world that are grounded in love, kindness, and compassion as opposed to aggression, criticism, and self-destruction.

Fortunately for us, learning to love ourselves unconditionally is not only possible, it's also a necessary, natural progression in both the biological and genetic evolution of humanity, as well as in the evolution of human consciousness globally. This means that life, nature, God, and the entire universe are all working with us, supporting us, and guiding us toward nothing less than total mastery over life's most empowering and most liberating lesson.

As you'll come to see, *You Were Not Born to Suffer* does not "beat around the bush." The pages that follow were intentionally written to guide you through an inner process that will empower you to completely change your life in ways that you cannot even begin to imagine.

Each chapter offers you practical guidance designed to create new, healthy neurological and energetic pathways within your mind and body, so you may begin to channel your thoughts, emotions, words, and actions toward loving yourself in every moment, situation, and relationship. What your life looks and feels like one month, one year, and one decade from now will, however, depend entirely on how serious you are about healing yourself and fulfilling your life's purpose.

Please ask yourself, "Just how serious am I about transforming and releasing the core psychological and emotional blocks that are holding me back from creating everything that I truly want and need in my life right now? Am I finally ready to let go of the limiting beliefs, self-destructive conditions, and painful emotions that are weighing me down and sabotaging my natural health, wealth, and happiness?"

I love the old saying that goes, "If you give a man (or woman) a fish he will eat for a day, but if you teach him to fish he will eat for a lifetime." With this in mind, *You Were Not Born to Suffer* will teach you how to fish for yourself. Its aim is to empower you to lovingly nourish and feed your soul for all of eternity. If you are indeed serious about improving the quality of your health, your relationships, your finances, and your career right now, then this book will undoubtedly support you to take your life, your power, and your destiny back into your own hands so you can do just that.

There is no difficulty that enough love will not conquer. There is no disease that enough love will not heal. No door that enough love will not open. No gulf that enough love will not bridge. No wall that enough love will not throw down. And no sin that enough love will not redeem. It makes no difference how deeply seated may be the trouble. How hopeless the outlook. How muddled the tangle. How great the mistake. A sufficient realization of love will dissolve it all. And if you could love enough you would be the happiest and most powerful person in the world.

—EMMET FOX

SELF-LOVE, WORLD PEACE, AND YOU

As consciousness continues to evolve throughout humanity, each day more and more of us are answering the inner call to embody the changes that we want to see most in the world around us. Inherent within this organic evolution, many of us are awakening to the obligation we have, both to ourselves and to our world, to master loving ourselves unconditionally.

The simple truth is that if we do not love all of who we are today, as well as all of who we have been in the past, it is impossible for us to truly be at peace within ourselves or our lives. It is not until we consciously make the choice to relate to ourselves with unconditional love, kindness, and compassion in every moment, situation, and relationship that we finally find the lasting inner peace we're all looking for.

When it comes to our collective destiny as one human family to create peace on this planet, it is crucial to grasp the fact that if we do not have unconditional love, acceptance, forgiveness, compassion, and respect for ourselves, then we cannot offer these qualities to other people. However, as we intentionally cultivate these virtues within ourselves, we not only expand our capacity to relate to other people in the same conscious and kind ways, but we simultaneously deepen our own experiences of inner peace as well.

Eventually, it becomes obvious that finding balance and harmony in our own lives is impossible when we relate to ourselves fearfully, aggressively, and critically. It is an indisputable fact that if we do not live and act in the world from a place of unconditional love, kindness, and compassion for ourselves, we will just continue to live and act in ways that are not only destructive and painful for ourselves but that are also damaging for the entire world around us. Thus, collectively, the time has now come for each of us to master life's most healing and redeeming lesson.

HEAL YOURSELF NOW QUESTIONS

Following most of the chapters throughout this book you will find questions specifically designed to transform the core psychological and emotional blocks that are holding you back in life. These questions will assist you in liberating as well as igniting vital life force energies that are trapped in your body, heart, mind, and life so you may release whatever is obstructing the inner peace, health, happiness, fulfillment, and love that's already alive within you.

As you work through the Heal Yourself Now Questions, it will be tremendously helpful to write out your answers, because expressing your thoughts and feelings in this way will help you to honor and clarify what is true for you. It will also free the psychological, emotional, physical, and spiritual life force energies that have become stuck in your body and your life. Thus, I highly recommend that you purchase a journal or notebook to write in as you read the remainder of this book. The potential change and forward movement these questions can inspire is truly unlimited if you take them to heart.

LOVE YOURSELF NOW
AFFIRMATIONS

Following the Heal Yourself Now Questions, you will also find Love Yourself Now Affirmations following most chapters in this book. These practices will support you to consciously think, feel, and express positive, healthy, and high-vibrational thoughts, emotions, and words.

As I mentioned before, the Heal Yourself Now Questions will free vital life force energies that have become trapped in your body, heart, mind, and life. Once liberated, these energies are then available for you to channel toward thinking, feeling, speaking, and acting in ways that support you to create what you want and need most in your life right now.

With this in mind, I have found that working with the Love Yourself Now Affirmations directly after answering the confronting Heal Yourself Now Questions is a very effective way to break through the limiting beliefs and unhealthy thought patterns that are currently sabotaging your inner peace, health, happiness, fulfillment, and freedom.

Additionally, I highly recommend that you use the following practice with all of the affirmations contained in this book. To make doing this simple, I recommend marking the next page so you can refer back to it after reading each chapter. At this point it's not necessary to read the following page, unless of course you feel inspired to.

Working with Love Yourself Now Affirmations

With your eyes either open or closed, wherever you are, please say each affirmation one at a time. If you are alone and you would like to say them out loud, please do so. If you are around other people and feel more comfortable expressing them only to yourself, that is very effective too.

Either way, please feel your whole body as you express each affirmation. Please feel your feet, your legs, your belly, your chest, your back, your arms, your hands, your neck, and your head. Please take a few slow, deep breaths through your nose into your belly, and then imagine that you are speaking to every cell in your body. When you have an opportunity, please also try expressing these affirmations in front of a mirror while looking into your eyes. This is a very powerful way to heal yourself and your life.

Please also note any negative thoughts, emotions, or physical sensations that arise within you as reactions to the affirmations you express. These will represent your subconscious blocks to living a fully healthy and happy life. Once aware of these inner, self-imposed limitations you'll be empowered to love yourself and reaffirm the positive, healthy thought patterns necessary to harmonize the negative or toxic energies that are trapped in your mind and body.

Lastly, please consider that it takes a little time to create new, healthy neurological and energetic pathways. I like to compare this process to digging a new irrigation channel or riverbed. At first it might feel a little like manual labor, but eventually the pathway is created and the energy can flow freely and naturally in a way that supports you rather than sabotages you.

When you have been thinking in a certain manner for a long period of time, it requires commitment and practice to redirect your thoughts, words, and actions consistently in a positive, healthy direction. Thus, when you find yourself doubting or rejecting a positive affirmation please know that this reaction represents a part of your psyche, personality, or identity that's developed to protect you from feeling emotional pain. In other words, when it's hard to accept or feel what you're affirming to be true, please be kind to yourself and know that the part of you that's resisting represents a part of you that's still hurting.

In time, through being patient and compassionate with yourself, the positive affirmations offered throughout this book will help you to heal your heart and liberate your soul. So please do not give up.

USING THE WORD *GOD*

Using the word *God* can be a sensitive subject. It is a word that holds the power to create either separation and war or unity and peace. Thus, I feel it is important to clarify and define the meaning of the word *God* as it is used throughout this book.

As you read, please keep in mind that I respect each religious tradition and spiritual path. In my own life, I have found that (1) all religious and spiritual study eventually leads to love in various forms, and (2) the only barriers between one human being and another are the unhealed emotions in our hearts and the limiting beliefs we hold in our heads. These two realizations have shaped and inspired much of this book.

In using the term *God* throughout the following pages, I am referring to everything and everyone in the universe, including the space in which no physical forms of life and no physical objects exist. By this definition, God refers to the intelligence, awareness, source, love, and atomic energy from which all life and all physical forms of matter in the universe arise. From this perspective, God exists in all people, all things, and all space as the people, things, and space themselves. God, here, also represents the vast sea of unlimited potential and possibility to which all life and all physical forms of matter eventually return.

*I have found the paradox, that if you love until it hurts,
there can be no more hurt, only more love.*

—MOTHER TERESA

CHAPTER ONE

The Butterfly

*The Greek name for a butterfly is Psyche, and the same word means the soul.
There is no illustration of the immortality of the soul so striking and beautiful
as the butterfly, bursting on brilliant wings from the tomb in which it has
lain, after a dull, grovelling, caterpillar existence, to flutter in the blaze of
day and feed on the most fragrant and delicate productions of spring. Psyche,
then, is the human soul, which is purified by sufferings and misfortunes,
and is thus prepared for the enjoyment of true and pure happiness.*

—BULFINCH'S MYTHOLOGY: THE AGE OF FABLE

The lifecycle of a butterfly is a perfect example found in nature that mirrors back to us what it means to break free from the limitations and fears that restrict us from living our most liberated and joyful life. The caterpillar's metamorphosis into a butterfly beautifully demonstrates the natural rhythms and processes of inner and outer transformation experienced by all life. In its physical form, the butterfly itself symbolizes the potential freedom and lightheartedness that are available to each and every one of us. Just seeing a butterfly reawakens us to the magic and wonder inherent in life. Its grace and vulnerability immediately take us beyond thought into the mystery of our own existence.

The butterfly begins its journey as a caterpillar, and it may or may not be aware of what it is destined to become. But the caterpillar lives on, faithfully following the inner prompts arising within its being. It *feels* its way through life, naturally following the inner direction with

1

which it was born. The caterpillar follows what seems to be an inner plan, which from the outside can be observed as inspiring the journey from caterpillar to cocoon and from cocoon to butterfly. The feeling and the pull into what appears to be the unknown must be so clear and so strong for the caterpillar, because when the time comes to create a cocoon for itself, in which both its inner and outer transformations will occur, the caterpillar carries out its intended purpose with a one-pointed focus and determination.

The caterpillar appears to feel that it does not have a choice but that it must surrender and follow the forces of nature and the universe as they propel and guide it forward, no matter what the journey entails. Once transformation is complete, the butterfly struggles with all of its strength to emerge from its cocoon. Eventually it leaves behind the protective shell that no longer serves any purpose. The butterfly's new existence only slightly resembles its old form. It does not know itself anymore. Its past has been left behind, and the butterfly now experiences itself as something changed and new. It has been reborn. And now it is free.

Our own journey through life is like this as well. Like the caterpillar's journey into its cocoon and its struggle to emerge as a butterfly, our own journey as human beings toward our most liberated and joyful life is one in which we also struggle to live gracefully and intentionally as a free and full expression of who and what we truly are. We all struggle to liberate ourselves from our suffering and thus free ourselves from our protective cocoon in order to embody the highest form of our own soul's evolution.

Within each one of us, there lives a sense of an inner plan that is always inspiring us to break free into the mystery of our existence. We too have this inner guidance directing us forward, a felt force deep within our soul propelling us onward in faith. Just like the butterfly that struggles to break free from the restricting confines of its cocoon, deep down our souls too know and trust that our own struggles will eventually open to the richness, wonder, and beauty of our most liberated and joyful life.

Ultimately, the struggle to liberate ourselves fully is the struggle to love ourselves unconditionally in every moment, situation, and relationship. In order to do this we're all called to consciously heal our psychological and emotional pain in the present. We're faced with the task of freeing ourselves from the protective cocoon that we've developed over time—this psychic shell that's been protecting us until we're ready to live our lives authentically and openheartedly as a free and full expression of who and what we truly are.

Just like the butterfly, the development of our own cocoon is natural and vital for our soul's evolutionary unfolding. Our cocoon serves us while we heal and go through the inner transformations necessary to fully embody our soul's true nature. At some point in our lives, however, our cocoon always becomes limiting and unhealthy. Once we've gone through the initial stages of healing and growth within the safety of this protective shell, all of us are called to liberate ourselves from a way of being in the world that no longer serves us.

When this time comes will vary for each of us, but it does indeed come. And when it does we're all faced with a life-defining choice. We either surrender and align with the forces of nature and the universe that are evolving within and through us or, we resist this evolutionary force and thereby create more struggle and pain for ourselves.

With this in mind, I'd like to share a touching story that I once read about a woman who brought two butterfly cocoons into her home that were about to hatch. The woman wanted to observe the butterflies break free from their cocoons and eventually take flight.

For days she eagerly watched, waiting for the butterflies to emerge. In time, she was able to witness one of the butterflies begin creating a small hole in its cocoon. From the woman's perspective, this first butterfly seemed to struggle painfully as it slowly pushed its way through the opening it had created. Once it was fully liberated, the butterfly lay there on the table, exhausted and unable to go any further. However, after a short period of time, the butterfly finally raised itself up and flew out a nearby window, fluttering on its strong and beautiful wings.

After observing the challenging process that the first butterfly experienced, the woman felt inspired to help the second butterfly free itself from its cocoon so it wouldn't have to struggle like the first one did. Meaning well, the woman decided to use a razor blade to gently slice down the center of the second butterfly's cocoon as it began its journey toward its liberation. Once freed, the second butterfly lay there on the table just like the first one did. However, after that same short period of time, rather than raising itself up and flying away, the second butterfly quietly died.

Confused about what had occurred, the woman contacted a friend who was a biologist and asked her to explain why the second butterfly had died. Her friend expressed that the challenging struggle the butterfly undergoes to liberate itself from its cocoon actually forces liquids from deep inside its body cavity out into the tiny capillaries in the butterfly's wings. This process is what causes a butterfly's wings to harden, making them strong enough and healthy enough for their new life of flight. She explained that without the struggle a butterfly experiences in breaking through its own cocoon, there could be no strength in its wings, no flight, and ultimately no life.

Just like the butterflies in this story, you and I are destined to liberate ourselves from the bonds of our own protective cocoons. And just like the caterpillar, we each have everything that we need within ourselves to (1) love ourselves unconditionally and (2) create the inner and outer freedom that we all intuitively desire.

When we stop to reflect on the deeper meaning of the above story we are graced with one of life's most beautiful and empowering lessons: *Each of us already has everything we need within ourselves to fulfill our life's purpose and realize our greatest potential. God, or the intelligent universe, created life this way. Life itself inherently holds all that it needs within itself to fully become all that it is destined to be. Our greatest potentials and strengths already live within us, just waiting to be cultivated and expressed fully in our lives.*

Unfortunately, however, too many of us live our whole lives without realizing this. We go through life living in fear, constantly relating to our world from the familiarity, comfort, and safety of our protective cocoon. Way too often we end up settling for a limited way of life, having never realized nor expressed the fullness or the greatness of who and what we all truly are.

If we don't just settle for cold comfort, a large majority of us continually search outside of ourselves, thinking that something or someone outside of us will free us. Maybe someone will rescue us or save us from the restricting confines of our own cocoon? Maybe someone will love us enough or care for us enough to liberate us from our personal struggles and make everything okay?

What an illusion this truly is!

All of us are born caterpillars in this life, and we all create a cocoon for ourselves as we grow. What differs among us, however, is that some of us are willing to follow the inner prompts of our heart and soul to become the liberated, passionate, and purposeful beings that we're destined to be, and some of us quite simply are not.

There seem to be only two options in life. We either become the butterfly that we're destined to be, or we don't. We either master loving ourselves unconditionally, and in so doing free ourselves from our cocoon, or we don't.

In the first option we undoubtedly struggle; sometimes we struggle deeply and it's painful. But with the struggle and the pain always come the magic, wonder, and beauty of living our most liberated and joyful life. The struggle and pain actually become worth it because we're blessed to experience the inherent freedom and joy of our soul's deepest and truest nature. We get to be free, and one could say that our soul gets to fly.

In the second option we either settle for the unconscious, fear-based comfort of our cocoon, or we wait for someone or something to come along and free us. We might live our whole lives waiting for someone to slice open our cocoon for us. In both cases, we end up living our entire lives unaware that we already have everything we need within us to liberate ourselves and to live the magnificent lives that we're all destined to live.

When we take this second path in life we remain trapped in our frustration and misery, and eventually our bodies stop functioning before we ever realize or express our inherent greatness. In this lifetime, we unconsciously pass up the magic, wonder, and beauty of living our most liberated and joyful life.

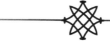

In the same way it is often said that the unexamined life is not worth living, I believe that a life without learning to love ourselves unconditionally is similarly not worth living. If you're honest with yourself in reading this, I'm sure you would agree that the pain, suffering, and confusion that result from an aggressive, fear-based, and self-destructive relationship with yourself makes life quite miserable and hardly worth living at times.

Considering this, loving ourselves unconditionally always leads to the lasting inner peace, health, happiness, and fulfillment we're all looking for. I have found that once we're finally ready to welcome and love all of who we are today, as well as all of who we have been in the past, we naturally find the strength, courage, and love within us that's necessary to heal ourselves, fulfill our life's purpose, and realize our greatest potential both personally and professionally.

I often ask myself: why would anyone settle for anything less?

What do you think?

CHAPTER TWO

The Purpose of Suffering

The world breaks everyone, and afterward, some
are strong at the broken places.

—ERNEST HEMINGWAY

> *Wherever you are, please take a few slow, deep breaths into*
> *your belly. Please also feel your whole body, from your feet all*
> *the way up to the crown of your head, and then down to your*
> *fingertips. Please surrender fully and accept everything that*
> *you're thinking, feeling, and experiencing here in this moment.*
> *Please be present to your body and your breath.*

E ven if we cannot see it, and even if we won't allow ourselves to
believe it, there is a much healthier, happier, and more peaceful
way of life waiting for all of us beyond the aspects of ourselves and our
lives that we're currently struggling with. Quite simply, you and I were
not born to suffer. Nor were we born to settle for anything less than a
truly passionate, purposeful, and fulfilling experience of life. You and
I were actually born to enjoy the gift of being human. We were born
to learn, to grow, to create beauty, to live our lives to the fullest, and
ultimately, to bring unconditional love abundantly into this world.

The single most important key to finding lasting inner peace, health,
happiness, and fulfillment in our lives is the realization that all of our

suffering is simply a cry from the depths of our soul, from who we truly are, asking us to love ourselves unconditionally in every moment, situation, and relationship. In other words, all the psychological, emotional, physical, financial, and spiritual struggle, pain, or illness that we experience is purely our soul's way of waking us up to the aspects of ourselves, our lives, and our past that we do not love fully here and now.

In essence, our suffering forces us to bring more awareness into our daily lives so we may master living with unconditional love, kindness, and compassion for ourselves, for other people, and for all life. Our suffering actually reawakens us to who and what we truly are so we may transform the unconscious aspects of ourselves and our lives that do not support our overall wellbeing or self-actualization.

Our internal and external struggles ultimately help us to learn the lessons beneath what we see as our "mistakes" in life. They help us to change, to grow, to evolve, and to thrive so we may come to live our lives in conscious ways that create less suffering and more harmony, not only for ourselves, but also for everyone around us.

Suffering is just a part of human life. It always has been and to some degree it always will be. Pain is how we truly learn to love ourselves and enjoy the life we've been given. It's also how we bring the unconditional love that we are fully into being. Even though life will always present us with challenges, once we're finally ready to face our deepest inner truths, we all can, and eventually we all will, transform the root causes of our suffering and find the lasting joy, freedom, and fulfillment that we're looking for.

> *No one decides against his happiness, but he*
> *may do so if he does not see he does.*
>
> —A COURSE IN MIRACLES

The inner restlessness, anxiety, confusion, sadness, depression, dissatisfaction, frustration, anger, hurt, resentment, fear, shame, guilt, regret, insecurity, inadequacy, self-judgment, and self-doubt that so many of us live with and struggle with on a daily basis are all merely the result of us not loving ourselves unconditionally throughout our lives. All the pain we've ever felt, all the pain we may feel now, and all the pain we will ever feel in our body, heart, or mind has its roots in all the times in the past where we have not loved, honored, and valued ourselves, but rather compromised, betrayed, abandoned, judged, rejected, and therefore hurt ourselves.

Only through accepting this universal truth and then applying it to our daily lives can we finally free ourselves from our suffering and create the healthy, happy, and fulfilling lives that we all deserve. Rather than relating to ourselves and talking to ourselves in the hard and aggressive ways that most of us currently do, we're all destined to ease up on ourselves and give ourselves the unconditional love, kindness, and compassion that we each need to thrive.

Would you agree that life is challenging enough without us being our own worst enemies?

There is no coming to consciousness without pain. People will do anything, no matter how absurd, in order to avoid facing their own soul. One does not become enlightened by imagining figures of light, but by making the darkness conscious.

—CARL JUNG

In mastering an unconditional love for ourselves, we're called to face ourselves and our lives honestly without running from or avoiding anyone or anything. Rather than becoming stuck in or identified with our life struggles, each of us is destined to view these apparent obstacles as empowering lessons to be learned and then courageously face them head on.

Unfortunately, however, many of us live our whole lives trapped in and consumed by our suffering because we constantly run from, avoid, and deny the things in ourselves, our lives, and our past that seem too painful or too scary to honestly address, feel, and embrace. Rarely are we taught that through honestly attending to these inner battles we can transform them, find peace, strength, and happiness within them, and ultimately move forward and thrive because of them. Most of us never realize that simply through facing our internal and external life challenges directly right here in the present moment we can heal their root causes and find lasting freedom from them.

Regardless of how much we try to avoid our pain and confusion in the present it will always remain repressed and stuffed deep down inside of us. And this denied psychological, emotional, physical, and spiritual pain not only makes us sick, miserable, and poor, it also causes us to react to life in ways that sabotage us and keep us stuck in the very situations, relationships, and self-destructive patterns that do not support our wellbeing or reflect who we truly are.

Only through consciously facing, feeling, and therefore healing all the uncomfortable and painful aspects of ourselves, our lives, and our past can we hear the life-changing messages and learn the liberating lessons buried within these challenges. No matter how painful, scary, or overwhelming they may be, each thought, emotion, and life experience is ultimately guiding our inner evolution toward complete self-healing, self-mastery, and self-realization. Every single situation and relationship—past, present, and future—is leading us toward an unconditional love for ourselves and toward the psychological, emotional, physical, financial, and spiritual freedom that we already know to be our destiny and our birthright.

The body's suffering is a mask the mind holds up to hide what really suffers.

—*A Course In Miracles*

Most of us were never taught that there is an ocean of pure love, joy, fulfillment, and peace buried beneath our suffering that is so plentiful words could never do justice in expressing this deep inner truth. Thankfully, as we intentionally transform our self-destructive relationship with ourselves into one that is always loving, kind, and compassionate, we cannot help but reconnect with this ever-present source that's already alive within each of us.

Once we've suffered enough to finally value ourselves and honor the evolutionary call of our soul asking us to love ourselves unconditionally in every moment, situation, and relationship, we'll always find that the love within us will both heal us and fulfill us completely from the inside out. In fact, the more we love ourselves, the more we realize that our suffering exists merely to guide us toward the amazing healthy and happy lives that we're all destined to live.

Heal Yourself Now Questions

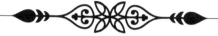

In what ways are you struggling within
yourself and your life right now?

What physical symptoms or illnesses is your body expressing
as a way of asking you to love yourself more fully?

What do you struggle to love about yourself here in the present?

What do you struggle to love about your life here in the present?

What do you struggle to love about yourself
and your life from the past?

Do you ever think about killing yourself? If so, why?

Are you aware that you'll just have to come back, or be reborn,
to face the same pain and to learn the same lessons?

What can you focus your energy on today that represents
you loving and valuing yourself and therefore honoring
what you love to do, want to do, or need to do?

Love Yourself Now Affirmations

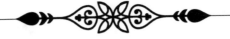

I was not born to suffer.

Today is the first day of the rest of my life.

I do not need to be sick to be loved.

Suicide will not solve my problems. Only love will.

It's never too late to start over. I can recreate my life.

There is a healthy and happy life waiting for me beyond my suffering.

I am not just my thoughts or my emotions. I am so much more.

The voice in my head is only a small part of me.

I have everything I need within me to be
healthy, happy, fulfilled, and free.

I am willing to master loving myself unconditionally.

This love inside of me will heal me and fulfill me completely.

I am grateful for my strong immune system,
and I thank it for protecting me.

There's no need for my body to get sick or age
because every cell is eternally self-healing. I love
myself daily, and so there's no need to suffer.

For the first time in my life I saw the truth as it is set into song by so many poets, proclaimed as the final wisdom by so many thinkers. The truth—that love is the ultimate and the highest goal to which man can aspire. Then I grasped the meaning of the greatest secret that human poetry and human thought and belief have to impart: The salvation of man is through love and in love. I understood how a man who has nothing left in this world still may know bliss, be it only for a brief moment, in the contemplation of his beloved. In a position of utter desolation, when man cannot express himself in positive action, when his only achievement may consist in enduring his sufferings in the right way—an honorable way—in such a position man can, through loving contemplation of the image he carries of his beloved, achieve fulfillment. For the first time in my life I was able to understand the meaning of the words, "The angels are lost in perpetual contemplation of an infinite glory."

—Viktor Frankl, Nazi concentration camp
survivor, *Man's Search for Meaning*

CHAPTER THREE

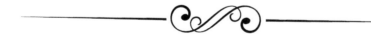

The Search for Love

The hunger for love is much more difficult to remove than the hunger for bread.

—MOTHER TERESA

Wherever you are, please take a few slow, deep breaths into your belly. Please also feel your whole body, from your feet all the way up to the crown of your head, and then down to your fingertips. Please surrender fully and accept everything that you're thinking, feeling, and experiencing here in this moment. Please be present to your body and your breath.

The search for love is the driving force behind everything that we do and everything that we desire in life. Whether it's a conscious process or not, we're all simply looking for love, because when it comes down to it, what else really matters? Once our basic survival needs for food, water, and shelter have been met, our need for love always surfaces as the sole motivating factor in life, because love is what heals us, fulfills us, and liberates our soul. Love alone creates beauty in the world, unlocks joy in our hearts, and makes life truly worth living. That's why, whether we're aware of it or not, every single one of us is either directly or indirectly in the pursuit of love right now.

Everything that we desire in life is born from this driving force of love within the depths of our heart and soul. And this universal desire for love that we all share is a deep longing within each of us to remember and embody our soul's deepest and truest nature—a nature that is, always has been, and always will be an infinite source of pure unconditional love.

Nearly all of us do what we do on a daily basis either because we want others to love us or because we want to love ourselves more fully. Until we awaken to the source of love within us, we all look for others to love us, because we haven't learned how to love ourselves yet. Paradoxically, it is our lack of love for ourselves in the present that keeps us from realizing that there already is an infinite source of pure unconditional love within the depths of our very own being.

As we come to love ourselves unconditionally, however, we fill ourselves up with the love that we seek while we simultaneously uncover the love that we are. And as we learn to relate to ourselves with unconditional love, kindness, and compassion in every moment, situation, and relationship, we also grow in our ability to embody love and thus give love back to life, which, in the end, is the highest expression of our soul's destiny and purpose in life.

Your task is not to seek for love, but merely to seek and find all the barriers within yourself that you have built against it.

—JALAL UDDIN RUMI

In our quest for healing, truth, happiness, and freedom, each of us is ultimately just looking for love. Life really is that simple. All of us search the outer world for what lives and has its home right in our very own hearts. Each and every one of us simply wants to be seen, understood, accepted, appreciated, valued, and loved unconditionally, just as we are. We all want to feel that our lives really matter, that we're not alone, and that even just one other person actually cares about our desires, our needs, our wounds, and our dreams.

The funny thing about us human beings is that love is the one thing we all want and need more than anything in life, and it's also the one thing that scares us more than anything else. Love scares us to our core because it requires our hearts to be open and vulnerable to ourselves, to other people, and to the world. We fear this love that we desire so deeply because it opens our hearts to life, and when our hearts are truly open and vulnerable we feel ourselves, we feel others, we feel our world, and we feel the love and the pain that we've held in, closed our eyes to, and disconnected from for so long.

Rather than fully feel the intensity of this sacred gift that we call life, the larger majority of us unintentionally close our hearts and cut ourselves off from the pulsating truth of what we feel because we're scared of experiencing the sometimes painful or uncomfortable emotions that are inherent to human existence. Of course, we're not aware of this, but in doing so we reject the infinite source of love within us and deny ourselves access to the one thing we desire above all else in life.

We're interesting creatures, aren't we?

Fortunately, the love alive within each of us is so powerful and so unstoppable that it will eventually heal and embrace every internal and external obstacle that stands in its way. The evolutionary impulse of life, nature, and the entire universe will always prevail in making sure that we fulfill our destiny to embody the love that we are.

As we allow ourselves to open to this deep inner truth, which happens to be truer than anything else we can know, feel, or say about ourselves, our lives immediately change for the better. We live each day knowing that we do not need to be more, do more, or have more to finally be loveable to ourselves or to others, because we've remembered that we are, and always have been, both loveable and abundant in love just the way we are.

> *Ask, and it will be given to you; seek, and you will find; knock,*
> *and it will be opened to you. For everyone who asks receives, and*
> *he who seeks finds, and to him who knocks it will be opened.*

> —MATTHEW 7:7–8

In the most down-to-earth, rational, logical, scientific, serious, and practical way that it's possible to express this deep truth and fact, I have found that our true nature, our soul, our spirit, who we really are, already is an infinite source of pure unconditional love.

With this in mind, please ask yourself the following questions.

1) Why would love ever need to search outside of itself for love?
2) How could love truly not love itself?

And yet we all do it. We're all like cute little puppy dogs chasing our tails.

The empowering, liberating, and healing reality, however, is that none of us need to search for love outside of ourselves at all, because we already have all the love we could ever want or need within us right now. We've all merely forgotten who and what we truly are, but the time has now come for each of us to remember once again.

Heal Yourself Now Questions

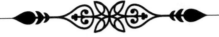

What do you love most in life and about life?

What are all of the little things and the big things that you love?

What are your favorite things to do, see, taste, touch,
smell, experience, feel, create, or accomplish?

What makes you happy?

What activities bring out your happiness?

What has made you happy in the past?

Whom do you love in your life? Whom do
you truly care about and value?

What would you say are your gifts and talents?

What are your "inner jewels" and strengths as a person?

Whom do you expect to make you happy or satisfy you?

Whose love, acceptance, approval, attention, recognition, emotional
support, or financial support do you seek on a regular basis?

Whom do you constantly try to please, make happy, or satisfy?

What would happen if you stopped?

What can you focus your energy on today that represents
you loving and valuing yourself and therefore honoring
what you love to do, want to do, or need to do?

Love Yourself Now Affirmations

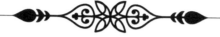

I am pure, unconditional love.

My soul is made of pure love.

There is an ocean of love inside of me.

I am one with the infinite universe.

I do not need to search outside of myself for love.

I am enough.

I am loveable just as I am.

I do not need to be more, do more, or have more
to love myself or to be loved by others.

God lives in me, as me.

I am the love of God.

CHAPTER FOUR

Start Honoring and Valuing Yourself Now

The hardest challenge is to be yourself in a world where
everyone is trying to make you be somebody else.

—E. E. CUMMINGS

> *Wherever you are, please take a few slow, deep breaths into*
> *your belly. Please also feel your whole body, from your feet all*
> *the way up to the crown of your head, and then down to your*
> *fingertips. Please surrender fully and accept everything that*
> *you're thinking, feeling, and experiencing here in this moment.*
> *Please be present to your body and your breath.*

It's often not until we allow other people to treat us horribly and therefore feel worthless or valueless that we realize our approach to ourselves and to life truly needs to change. Unfortunately, things have to get so bad, so painful, or so out of control for most us before we realize how important it is to honor and value ourselves consistently in every moment, situation, and relationship.

For those of us who never learned to love ourselves, and for those of us who often feel inadequate, insecure, underserving, or unworthy of love, we will constantly abandon and betray ourselves for the love of others to the point where we repeatedly find ourselves in situations and relationships where we feel used, unappreciated, valueless, or worthless to those around us as well as to ourselves.

Underneath these painful situations and relationships, however, is the empowering and healing truth that we're not actually victims in any way, because we're the ones who have compromised ourselves for the conditional love, acceptance, approval, attention, and support of other people and thus can change this self-destructive pattern.

If we look at ourselves honestly, most of us will see that we often do not honor and value what we truly think, feel, want, and need, because we're afraid to, we don't know how to, or we don't feel that we deserve to. In other words, we all compromise ourselves to varying degrees on a daily basis just to "keep the peace" and to avoid confrontation. Some of us compromise ourselves in every situation and relationship because we unconsciously believe that we must always please others or make others happy in order to be loved, accepted, approved of, attended to, or supported. Some of us don't compromise ourselves nearly as much but still find it challenging at times to love, honor, and value ourselves fully.

What most of us don't realize until we've allowed our own sense of self-worth and self-respect to reach zero is that in every moment, situation, and relationship that we do not honor and value ourselves, we are compromising who we really are and thus abandoning, betraying, and ultimately hurting ourselves far more deeply than we know. This hurt that we all unconsciously inflict upon ourselves when we disregard our inner truths then creates deep anger, frustration, resentment, hatred, and dissatisfaction within us that we hold toward ourselves—and this self-destructive dynamic occurring within each of us is actually the root cause of all the anger and hatred that exists in our world.

Knowing this, in every moment of every day we are either loving, honoring, and valuing ourselves or, we are compromising, abandoning, and hurting ourselves. In each moment, situation, and relationship that we allow our fears of losing love, acceptance, approval, attention, security, or support to determine our choices and actions, we add to the buildup of pain, anger, misery, and inner dis-ease that we've already created for ourselves by compromising and betraying ourselves so much throughout our lives. On the other hand, in each moment, situation, and relationship that we face our fears and thus choose to love, honor, and value ourselves come what may, we heal our suffering in the present and we move forward into the psychological, emotional, physical, financial, and spiritual freedom that is our birthright.

Underneath all of the situations and relationships in which we currently compromise ourselves there is simply a very old and deep survival fear operating that has its roots in our early years as children. Growing up, most of us never felt safe enough to fully be ourselves or to express everything that we felt, thought, wanted, or needed. As a result, our instincts led all of us to compromise, abandon, fragment, and betray ourselves in exchange for the conditional love, approval, acceptance, attention, security, and support that we felt we needed from our parents, our teachers, our peers, and our caregivers just to survive. These old and deep fears that we all carry to some degree then lead each of us to compromise and betray ourselves throughout our adult lives. Whether it's with our parents, our children, other family members, our spouses, our partners, our friends, our colleagues, our employers, or our employees, most of us still abandon our inner truths in exchange for something.

This soul-destroying exchange might come in the form of love, acceptance, attention, approval, safety, security, or some kind of support. It may also come in the form of money, fame, vanity, companionship, pleasure, or sex. Regardless of who or what we've compromised ourselves for over the years, the truth is that many of us have created a completely compromised life because we haven't learned to break through our fears of losing love and security to always honor and value who we genuinely are. Consequently, this unconscious fear for our survival, which most of us will recognize quite easily within ourselves, constantly sabotages our natural health, wealth, and happiness until we're able to consciously face it and choose to love ourselves unconditionally regardless of what it entails.

Both in myself and in my private practice I've seen one common reason why so many of us continue to compromise ourselves for the love, acceptance, approval, and support of other people: *we do not feel that we are loveable or deserving of love just the way we are.* This particular dynamic drives many of us to stay in situations, relationships, and jobs that do not reflect our deepest inner truths, ultimately because we hold the destructive belief that no one else will stand by us, love us, or employ us if we truly honor and value ourselves.

Way too many of us live believing that we lack something within ourselves, which renders us unlovable or undeserving of the love, happiness, respect, and fulfillment we all deserve. Even though this is completely untrue, we still end up hurting ourselves because we feel the only way to be loved, accepted, approved of, or supported by another person, by other people, or by a business is to please them and make them happy, even if it's at the expense of our own integrity, health, happiness, or well-being.

This self-destructive pattern of relating to ourselves is created very early in our lives, and most of us just live out the majority of our days "prostituting" ourselves and disregarding both our own values and our own needs for this tainted love, acceptance, approval, and support from other people. As a result, our lives become a constant struggle to please others while deep down we remain tense, unhappy, and unsatisfied. What we fail to realize is that simply by loving, honoring, and valuing ourselves in each moment, situation, and relationship, starting now, we can heal our inadequacies and insecurities and thereby discover that we've always been abundant and deserving in every way imaginable.

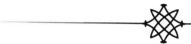

Learning to love and honor the very deepest parts of ourselves is often a painful stage in our awakening through which we finally claim the intrinsic value and worth of our lives in and of themselves. Thus, regardless of how it appears from the outside, we all live with parts of ourselves that are like dark rooms in which fragments of our soul feel mistreated or abandoned, and it seems as though no one is listening to our pain-filled cries. Ironically, it is we ourselves whom we're calling out to, asking our higher selves to turn on the lights and flood these dark spaces within us with a deep self-love and respect.

When we've lived believing and feeling that we're not loveable or deserving of love just as we are, we find that there exist a number of these "dark rooms" or "blind spots" within us that are devoid of self-value and self-worth. As we touched on before, it's often not until we allow ourselves to be used or taken advantage of that we realize that we're in fact the ones who have somehow betrayed ourselves.

When this is the case, as it is for the majority of us, we purposefully create situations and experiences where we invite people into our lives to exploit us and thus reveal the wounded parts of ourselves that are still hurting and waiting to be rescued with self-love. Through our quest for peace, health, happiness, and fulfillment our soul is calling us home, asking us to turn on the lights in these parts of ourselves so we can assert from deep inside our being that *we do not want to create any more suffering for ourselves.* Once we finally make this assertion, the courage arises within us to stand strong and flood these once darkened spaces with a knowing that we deserve genuine love, kindness, and respect in every aspect of our lives.

It's helpful to know that these parts of ourselves that are temporarily devoid of light and love are the sole causes for the relationships and situations in our lives where we do not feel honored, valued, or respected by other people. With this in mind, once we commit to enlightening these painful, love-deprived spaces within us, we're also called to stick up for our inherent value and worth in every aspect of our personal and professional lives. This unavoidable process of recreating our inner relationship with ourselves is often one of the most difficult aspects of our ongoing healing and spiritual journey, because it requires us to value ourselves enough to either recreate or leave behind every situation that does not mirror back our newfound self-respect and self-worth.

As our love for ourselves grows, we're repeatedly challenged to look at our personal and professional lives and to ask ourselves, "Where and with whom am I allowing myself to be mistreated, disrespected, or unappreciated? Where are these dark rooms in which my soul is crying out for my protection, strength, and love? When will I finally reach the point where l proclaim, 'Enough misery, enough living a lie, and enough settling for less than I know I'm worthy, deserving, and capable of!'?"

As we mature spiritually, emotionally, and psychologically it's also important to understand that when we compromise our inner truths for any reason, what we say and how we act do not represent what we truly believe, think, feel, want, or need. When we fail to honor and value ourselves in any scenario, our inner world becomes fragmented, confused, and imbalanced, because we've created an inner battle between who we really are and our fear-based compromises. In mastering an unconditional love for ourselves, however, our intention is to integrate and align our beliefs, thoughts, emotions, actions, and spoken words in every single moment, because this inner unity is what heals our pain and creates peace, health, joy, fulfillment, connection, ease, and love both within us and within our lives.

From a larger perspective, the more aligned we are internally, the more aligned we become externally with all of life, nature, and the entire universe. And when we live in such a state of internal alignment, the infinite universe is able to flow through us without getting stopped by the psychological, emotional, and physical blockages created when we abandon, betray, and hurt ourselves. As we master honoring and valuing ourselves in every moment, situation, and relationship, therefore, we end up breaking through both the fear and the emotional pain that obstruct the natural force and flow of the universe, which is (1) always guiding us toward our destiny and full potential and (2) always providing us with the necessary strength and energy to consciously create what we want and need most in our lives.

On a practical level, honoring ourselves means saying no sometimes; it often means we hold strong, standing in our truth, and then face whatever reactions arise when we do not speak and act merely to please others or to make them happy. Sometimes valuing ourselves means that we need to leave a relationship, a job, or a certain place, knowing deep down that our daily health, happiness, and fulfillment are more important than the safety and security of cold, heartless, financial or material comfort.

Once we've suffered enough and are thus ready to honor and value ourselves without compromising our inner truths for anyone or anything, the universe will always step up to help us on our destined path. We cannot know exactly how God will conspire to provide us with precisely what we need to move forward and to thrive, but we can always be certain that we'll be supported in fulfilling our life's purpose to bring the unconditional love that we are fully into this world.

Ultimately, each day our commitment to ourselves and our faith in life are tested merely to show us the fear that still remains alive within us so we can transform it, heal it, and come to love ourselves and our lives more deeply. This process continually reveals the inner strength that we're all born with to fearlessly love, honor, and value ourselves in every moment, situation, and relationship, and in so doing create the liberated, joyful, and fulfilling life that we're all destined to live.

Heal Yourself Now Questions

Where and with whom in your life right now are you
compromising yourself and abandoning your inner truth,
in any way, for love, acceptance, approval, companionship,
emotional support, financial support, safety, or security?

Why are you compromising, abandoning, and betraying yourself?

With whom in your life do you struggle to say
no? Why do you struggle to say no?

Who in your life do you feel you must always
please, satisfy, or make happy?

Have you ever felt abandoned by anyone? If so, can you see
how you had abandoned yourself or your inner truth somehow
in the relationship? Can you see how this subconscious pattern
has most likely been recurring since your childhood?

Where in your life are you settling for less than you know you
are worthy, deserving, or capable of? Why are you settling?

What do you want and need for yourself and
your life that you're neglecting?

What can you do on a daily basis that represents you taking
the time to consistently honor, value, and love yourself?

Love Yourself Now Affirmations

I do not need to compromise myself for love.

It's okay for me to say no and to hold strong
on what I want and need for myself.

I do not need to be more, do more, or have
more for others to love me.

I am loveable just the way I am.

I am enough. I am not lacking in anything.

I deserve to be honored, valued, and appreciated.

I am worthy and deserving of love.

I will not settle for less than I am worthy, deserving, or capable of.

I will not abandon or betray myself ever again.

CHAPTER FIVE

Always Express Your Inner Truth

*Be who you are and say what you feel, because those who
mind don't matter and those who matter don't mind.*

—Dr. Seuss

*Wherever you are, please take a few slow, deep breaths into
your belly. Please also feel your whole body, from your feet all
the way up to the crown of your head, and then down to your
fingertips. Please surrender fully and accept everything that
you're thinking, feeling, and experiencing here in this moment.
Please be present to your body and your breath.*

Pretty much all of the psychological, emotional, and physical
suffering that you might be experiencing in your life right now has
its roots in all the times in the past where you did not honor, value, and
therefore express what you were truly thinking and feeling. Universally,
our unexpressed psychological and emotional pain becomes physical
pain and illness when it goes unprocessed and thus unhealed. In fact,
most of the physical diseases that we experience as human beings are
actually just the result of stressful, toxic thoughts and emotions that have
gone unexpressed for long periods of time. We're obviously not aware
of it, but when we do not express our inner truths because of who or

what we fear, we're actually creating serious pain, confusion, sickness, and misery both for ourselves and for our world.

When we do not honor and thus express what we think, feel, want, and need, the psychological, emotional, and physical life force energies within our body, heart, and mind cannot flow freely, which then causes all of the functions in our body to weaken and eventually break down. On top of this, any time that we repress, deny, or internalize what we think, feel, want, or need, we actually create anger, resentment, frustration, guilt, and shame within us that literally eats us alive.

Whenever we do not express our inner truths, for any reason, the life-giving emotional energy that is meant to flow freely through us and from us becomes depressed, stuck, and trapped. And, if this energy is not expressed over time, it slowly builds up within us, causing our blood and cells to stagnate, coagulate, and eventually become palpable physical blockages to the healthy flow of our spirit and life force (i.e. tumors, cysts, masses, nodules).

To make matters worse, these energies and emotions that we tend to internalize, deny, and repress are often toxic and painful, so if we have not learned to express and release them, they end up creating severe toxicity within our body, heart, and mind. Sticking up for ourselves, therefore, is one of the most effective and practical forms of preventative medicine available to us. Through expressing what we think and feel we keep our vital life force energy, blood, and spirit moving and flowing throughout our being, which naturally heals us and fulfills us on a continual basis.

From this perspective, it's easy to see how over time our habits of "shoving" what we feel clog up the various biological systems within us and weaken our cells' natural abilities to repair themselves and produce energy, health, and happiness. Additionally, in any moment, situation, or relationship that we do not express our inner truths, we once again hurt ourselves, which just creates more anger, resentment, and frustration within us toward ourselves.

In both the world of spirituality and in the world of holistic, complementary, and alternative medicines, it is a widely accepted fact that most forms of cancer in the human body have their roots in repressed psychological and emotional anger. With this in mind, it becomes quite clear that regularly expressing ourselves is not only an important factor in avoiding serious illness and disease, but it is also a key to maintaining optimal levels of health, well-being, and happiness psychologically, emotionally, and physically throughout our lives.

At the root of our unhealthy patterns of internalizing, denying, and repressing what we think and feel, we once again find the fact that most of us never felt safe or supported enough growing up to fully express ourselves. On a deeper level, we never learned how to be present to our inner world or how to verbalize what we truly felt, thought, desired, or needed at various stages throughout our childhood. In the same ways that we began to compromise, abandon, and betray ourselves as young children, we also began to repress, deny, and internalize our thoughts and feelings, because we feared the pain that we associated with losing the love, acceptance, approval, or support of our parents and caregivers.

What was even more disheartening for many of us was that when we did find the strength and courage to express ourselves in the best ways that we knew how, we were often met with either angry reactions or with complete indifference and disregard. This makes it easy to see how in addition to our fears of losing love, many of us developed a pattern of internalizing our thoughts, feelings, desires, needs, and dreams because it didn't seem to make a difference to anyone whether or not we spoke up. Thus, a number of us just gave up on expressing ourselves long before we were even equipped with the tools or the language to do so effectively.

Now, in reaction to these early experiences, most of us have lived our whole adult lives replaying these childhood patterns of relating to the people around us. To many of us here in the present it seems as though no one cares about what we think or feel when in reality we gave up on learning how to express ourselves clearly a long time ago. Ultimately, as "adults," if we want our feelings, thoughts, needs, desires, and dreams to matter to the people currently in our lives, these inner realities must first matter to us, regardless of how they're received. Each of us is called to honor and value everything that arises within us before we can create and attract people in our lives who genuinely want to understand us and know us at the depths of our heart and soul.

Regardless of our age or the stage of life we're presently in, internalizing, denying, and repressing what we think, feel, want, or need in any moment, situation, or relationship out of fear is one of the most unhealthy, aggressive, and self-destructive patterns of relating to ourselves that we hold. In order to maintain a healthy, balanced flow of energy and emotion in both our bodies and our lives, we have to learn to welcome all of what we think and feel and then express ourselves with awareness and personal responsibility.

Thus, to heal ourselves and fulfill our life's purpose, we are all challenged to consciously express our feelings, thoughts, needs, desires, and dreams without allowing our fears of losing love or upsetting others to stop us or hold us back. Even when we're feeling confused or unclear about how we feel in any given moment or situation, it's still better to open up and communicate our inner truths, because it's only through expressing ourselves that we find the clarity and understanding within ourselves that's necessary to move forward with awareness, peace, and love. Just like a rusty water faucet that hasn't been used for a long time, we have to flush out the blockages and muddled energies in our own expression channels before we can consistently communicate our thoughts and feelings in conscious, clear, and mutually respectful ways.

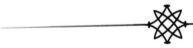

Learning to express ourselves fully also entails taking responsibility for how we react when we feel that we're not being heard. A number of us tend to yell and scream when we feel that what we're saying or trying to communicate is not being valued. So, in the aim of cultivating deep self-love and respect, we're faced with the task of mastering the process of expressing what we think and feel in nonviolent and unaggressive ways.

This task presents a deep challenge for many of us who grew up around people who used angry reactions and emotional manipulation as a means to control various situations and thus avoid taking personal responsibility. Learning to be accountable for what we think and feel while simultaneously expressing ourselves with awareness, respect, and love might be one of the most difficult lessons life presents to us, especially because we tend to take on the same unconscious patterns of emotional control and manipulation in our own lives that we were witness to growing up.

What's crucial to understand here is that underneath all the moments in which we feel the need to scream or yell to be heard, and underneath all the moments in which we've witnessed those we love and care about scream or yell to get a point across, the truth is that we're all hurting in our hearts and have never learned how to consciously express what we feel. Our angry reactions and the aggressive behaviors that result are merely our unconscious ways of protecting ourselves from past emotional pain that we've never felt safe enough or supported enough to feel and express, and in so doing heal.

To make matters worse, on top of never learning how to express ourselves in conscious and responsible ways, most of us learned a way of speaking to each other that is full of aggression, projection, and blame. Rather than learning the tools to consciously and respectfully say "I think," "I feel," "I want," or "I need" so and so, we learned to say things like "You" this or "You" that or "You're such a ..." or "You never ...," etc. In other words, we learned a form of communication that very effectively breeds hurt, defensiveness, and separation as opposed to open communication, trust, understanding, mutual respect, and deep connection.

The result of this painful cycle that's been passed down from generation to generation is people who are constantly crying out to be heard, valued, respected, and loved. Thankfully, however, there's a very simple solution to this very old and deep problem. All we have to do is awaken to the fact that we're not only one hundred percent responsible for what we think and feel, but we're also one hundred percent responsible for (1) valuing what we think and feel, and (2) expressing what we think and feel from a place of honesty, kindness, and respect.

If we can accept that underneath all our angry emotional reactions, both spoken and in thought, there's simply a part of us that's hurting and thus protecting us from further pain, we can choose to be courageous enough to face our hurting hearts and finally allow ourselves to heal the emotional and psychic wounds from our past. Ultimately, below every screaming match or aggressive form of communication, there's a little boy or little girl who's crying out for the unconditional love and support of his or her mother and/or father. When we can see ourselves and others in this penetrating light, we cannot help but open our hearts and express ourselves in kind, vulnerable ways that lead to healing, happiness, and connection instead of further pain and feelings of isolation.

Regardless of how much verbal abuse or aggression we've either witnessed or taken part in, deep down we all want to express ourselves clearly, lovingly, and consciously and feel that we're being heard, validated, and respected at each step along the way. We all want to feel that the people in our lives care enough to want to understand us in the depths of our heart and soul. What most of us fail to realize—and thus fail to take responsibility for—is that we ourselves have to care enough about ourselves to value, respect, and express what we're thinking, feeling, wanting, and needing before we can expect to create and attract relationships that consistently meet us in the deep ways we all intuitively desire and know that we deserve.

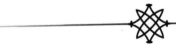

In the end, a very large part of our destiny and purpose in life is to consciously create our daily lives as an expression of the beauty and love within us. Achieving this is only possible through intentionally expressing the depths of our heart and soul in every moment, situation, and relationship, because through this process our outer reality increasingly reflects back to us the magnificent, compassionate, and harmonious vision of the world that's alive within each of us.

Ultimately our own voice is the voice of God, the voice of the intelligent universe expressing itself through our own unique lives as it guides us toward the inner peace, health, and happiness that we came here to enjoy. Our soul's true voice is also the voice of love, and it is this love that heals us and fulfills us, and then expands out to heal our loved ones and our world.

One could say that you and I are instruments in God's grand symphony orchestra, and we're all here to play an intentional part in the universe's creative masterpiece. From this perspective, each of us was born purposefully with an obligation to use our voice to stick up for what we know we came here to give, be, and do. Thus, we all have a responsibility not only to ourselves but also to each other to express our inner truths in the service of creating a world that is full of the kindness, respect, beauty, and love that we each hold abundantly within the depths of our heart and soul.

Heal Yourself Now Questions

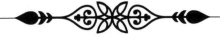

Where and with whom in your life do you struggle to express your inner truths? Where and with whom in your life right now do you struggle to express what you think, feel, want, and need?

Where and with whom in the past have you struggled to express your inner truths?

Who in your life right now do you fear being honest with? Are you afraid of upsetting them, hurting them, or losing their love and support?

What are you *feeling* right now about yourself and your life?

What do you truly *want* in your life right now, both internally and externally?

What do you *need* right now in your life?

Do you have anyone that you can *share* this with?

Love Yourself Now Affirmations

I express my truth and trust that all will be okay.

I forgive myself for not expressing myself in the past.

I do not need to fear punishment. I'm not a child anymore.

Expressing my emotions is the path to
health, happiness, and fulfillment.

I express my needs and desires with love, respect, and awareness.

What I feel, need, and want matters.

My voice is the voice of God and the voice of love.

Additional Practice for Self-Expression

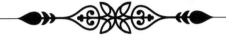

When you have time, please do yourself a favor and write letters to the people in your life, both past and present, whom you've never fully expressed yourself toward. Specifically writing one letter to your mother and one letter to your father is extremely healing and liberating. Other significant people include: children, partners, spouses, ex-partners, siblings, and friends.

At first, please write each letter as though you're not going to give the letter to the person so you may be completely honest with yourself about your feelings without holding anything back. Please keep in mind that it's okay, and also healthy, to express your anger as you write, because it's better to get this energy out than it is to keep it in. Later on, if you'd like to actually give a letter to any or all of these important people, you can write a less reactive form of the letter.

Also, if there are people in your life who have passed away whom you (1) never found closure with or (2) simply want to share things with, please also write them a letter. They can hear you and you can heal your pain if you express it and allow yourself to feel it.

CHAPTER SIX

Surrender Now and Let Go

*When you surrender to what is and so become fully present, the past
ceases to have any power. The realm of Being, which had been obscured
by the mind, then opens up. Suddenly, a great stillness arises within
you, an unfathomable sense of peace. And within that peace, there is
great joy. And within that joy, there is love. And at the innermost core,
there is the sacred, the immeasurable, That which cannot be named.*

—ECKHART TOLLE

---

*Wherever you are, please take a few slow, deep breaths into
your belly. Please also feel your whole body, from your feet all
the way up to the crown of your head, and then down to your
fingertips. Please surrender fully and accept everything that
you're thinking, feeling, and experiencing here in this moment.
Please be present to your body and your breath.*

Most of our suffering and unhappiness in life arise when we
resist or fight anything that we're feeling or anything that
we're experiencing in any given moment. Thus much of our healing
and happiness are found through accepting whatever we're feeling or
experiencing in each moment, situation, and relationship. When we stop
running from and resisting life in the here and now, we immediately
empower ourselves to see the thoughts, beliefs, and emotions, as well
as the situations and relationships, that are not grounded in a deep love

and respect for ourselves, ultimately so we can transform and heal these aspects of ourselves and our lives. Learning to let go and open fully to life in the present moment, therefore, is a key to identifying everything within us and within our lives that we're unconsciously allowing to limit us or hold us back.

To master loving ourselves unconditionally, and thus liberate ourselves from suffering, we are called to let go of our inner resistance to everything that we're not at peace, happy, or satisfied with in our lives, because it's only through complete inner acceptance that we can truly honor ourselves and redirect our life force energies toward creating what we want and need most to fulfill ourselves and our life's purpose.

Beneath our inner resistance to anyone or anything, we'll always find our fears of losing control, of losing our identity, of losing love, and ultimately of experiencing the unprocessed emotional pain that we've stored in our body, heart, and mind. In other words, underneath everything and everyone that we're reactive toward and feel somehow restricts our inner freedom, peace, or happiness, we're once again just protecting ourselves from feeling uncomfortable, scary, or overwhelming repressed emotions.

Ironically, the parts of ourselves and our lives that challenge us the most always represent the things we're most attached to and thus afraid of living without. In fact, whatever or whomever we grasp onto, to our own detriment, clearly shows us where we're still not fully loving, accepting, honoring, valuing, expressing, trusting in, or believing in ourselves.

Internally, we become attached to limiting beliefs about ourselves and the world ultimately because they protect us and distract us from facing what we fear feeling within ourselves and subconsciously know we need to heal. The same is also true for our self-destructive patterns of behavior as well as for our addictions. Beneath all of our habitual reactions, obsessions, and compulsions, all that exists are painful emotions that we haven't felt safe or supported enough to openly express or process.

Externally, we become attached to people, situations, jobs, money, and material possessions for the very same reasons. Underneath our attachments in the outer world, we always find the same fears of losing control, of losing our identity, of losing love, and ultimately of facing the uncomfortable emotions that we've denied and suppressed throughout our lives.

Thankfully, all of our attachments are connected to internal reactions purposefully designed first to protect us and then later to inspire our greatest psychological, emotional, physical, financial, and spiritual well-being. Our attachments, and the fear-coated emotions beneath them, actually show us exactly where we must surrender in our daily lives so we can let go of whatever or whomever we're still allowing to hold us back or drain our vital life force energy, health, and happiness.

If you realize that all things change, there is nothing you will try to hold on to. If you are not afraid of dying, there is nothing you cannot achieve.

—Lao Tzu

In learning to surrender fully we have no choice but to let go of our compulsive need to control ourselves, other people, and our environments, which means we must break through our fears of feeling the emotional pain that lives beneath our lack of openness, acceptance, and trust. No matter what we face in our outer life circumstances, learning to surrender fully without fighting anything or anyone, especially our own emotions and thoughts, is one of the most liberating lessons we're destined to learn on our healing and spiritual journey.

Regardless of how long we avoid addressing a particular issue, the time always comes when we cannot run from the truth any longer. At these points in our personal growth we realize that we have to accept the fact that we can only heal and change ourselves. Only we ourselves can take the necessary steps toward changing and growing in the direction of our destiny and our dreams. When these times inevitably arise, we're called to (1) stop trying to change other people, (2) stop trying to control the outside world, and (3) honor ourselves by following our hearts into the unknown territories and experiences that await us. We are challenged not to abandon our inner truths any longer but to break through our fears and self-imposed limitations to fulfill ourselves and the purpose of our lives.

Ultimately, there is nothing that we are not capable of transforming or recreating, so when we love ourselves enough to finally surrender our inner fight, we find that the love inside of us is strong enough to heal and transform anything that has been, or still is, painful or scary for us.

God, grant me the serenity to accept the things I cannot change, the courage to change the things I can, and the wisdom to know the difference.

—REINHOLD NIEBUHR

Everything in nature organically releases whatever limits its greatest potential for happiness, vitality, and life. In the same way many trees naturally let go of their leaves each autumn to make room for new growth and fresh life, so too are we destined to release the parts of ourselves, our lives, and our past that no longer serve our soul's growth and expansion. Since we are integral parts of nature, when we finally surrender to our soul's deepest inner calling, we too will freely let go of anything or anyone that we've allowed to limit us or hold us back in any way.

In learning to love ourselves unconditionally, we cannot allow ourselves to settle for anything less than our most liberated and joyful life, and this unfolding dynamic always entails letting go of the beliefs, habits, cold comforts, situations, and relationships that no longer reflect our soul's deepest inner truths. *Fortunately, as we focus on whom and what we love, follow our heart, and go after what we want and need most in life, we naturally leave behind everything that we do not want and everything that does not support our greatest health and happiness. Through loving, valuing, and honoring ourselves in every moment, situation, and relationship, everything that does not reflect who we truly are or why we're really here naturally just falls away, because life was perfectly designed to be this way.*

Just like the tree that is destined simply to be itself and to grow into a free and full expression of who and what it truly is, so too are we destined to love ourselves enough to live our lives as a free and full expression of who and what we truly are. Our tasks are simply to (1) surrender fully to whatever is true here and now, (2) let go of anxiously trying to control everyone and everything around us, (3) get crystal clear about what we want, need, and love, and (4) go after it with unwavering commitment, focus, and patience.

Heal Yourself Now Questions

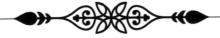

In which situations and relationships do you
find yourself constantly reacting?

Which people and environments do you struggle with and thus avoid?

Can you try to remain centered, present, and nonreactive
in these situations by breathing slowly and deeply?

Whom or what are you attached to and
intuitively know is holding you back?

Why are you afraid of moving on and letting
this person, situation, or thing go?

Whom in your life do you try to control? Your partner
or spouse? Your children or parents? Are you afraid
that they will abandon you or hurt you if you allow
them to do as they please? Why are you afraid?

Whom in your life do you feel controlled or dominated
by? Are you afraid of losing their love, upsetting them,
or being abandoned by them? Why are you afraid?

Are you attached to your material possessions? In other words, are
you afraid of losing any material object that you "own"? If so, why?

Do you identify with your material possessions?

Do you think they define who you are?

Can you name any belief or story you tell yourself that
you know limits you and holds you back in life?

What can you focus your energy on today that represents
you loving and valuing yourself and therefore honoring
what you love to do, want to do, or need to do?

Love Yourself Now Affirmations

I am whole, full, and complete.

I am willing to let go of my need to control
life. All control is an illusion.

I am willing to surrender my inner fight. I have suffered enough.

It's okay for me to let go and find peace.

My possessions cannot, do not, and will never define me.

I face my fears and move forward anyway.

I am okay, and I will be okay.

I am one with life. Everything is as it's meant
to be for my healing and growth.

(Your name), let go, let go, let go.

CHAPTER SEVEN

Take One Hundred Percent Personal Responsibility

When you think everything is someone else's fault, you will suffer a lot. When you realize that everything springs only from yourself, you will learn both peace and joy.

—His Holiness the 14ᵗʰ Dalai Lama

Wherever you are, please take a few slow, deep breaths into your belly. Please also feel your whole body, from your feet all the way up to the crown of your head, and then down to your fingertips. Please surrender fully and accept everything that you're thinking, feeling, and experiencing here in this moment. Please be present to your body and your breath.

Ultimately, by blaming other people, factors, or circumstances outside of ourselves for how we feel or for the life that we ourselves have created, we are giving away our personal power to create what we truly want and need most in our lives right now. If we sincerely want to free ourselves from our suffering, master loving ourselves unconditionally, and thereby create the passionate, purposeful, and fulfilling life that we're all destined to live, each of us is called to accept one hundred percent responsibility for our lives in their entirety.

If you're aware that you place blame outside of yourself for any reason, or that you play the victim sometimes with certain people, or in certain situations, please know that you're not alone. We all do it. All of us have played, or still play, the victim at times in our lives because it is the most common way that we've all learned to get what we want and need both from life and from other people.

If you imagine a small child who cries, throws a tantrum, or pouts to get his or her parents' attention, or to get what he or she wants and needs, you have a perfect example of what I mean. Now, please consider—and please also open to accepting the fact—that this same small child is most likely still very much alive inside of *you*, leading you to react and play the victim in your life, along with almost everyone else on our planet, including myself.

If we're honest with ourselves, many of us will see that we complain about or blame other people and factors outside of ourselves for the hurt, unhappiness, and dissatisfaction that we feel in relation to ourselves or our current life circumstances. This victim consciousness that so many of us live in is one of the most self-destructive and self-sabotaging belief patterns that we must transform within ourselves in order to (1) master loving ourselves unconditionally and (2) liberate ourselves from our suffering.

The "poor me" way of life that so many of us are trapped in to some degree ultimately keeps us stuck in the very situations and relationships in which we feel hurt and victimized. Thus, if we truly want to find lasting inner peace, health, happiness, and fulfillment, we must stop allowing ourselves to believe that we are, or ever have been, the victim in any way, at any point, in any situation or relationship.

The vulnerable truth is that at a very young age most of us learned that if we played the victim, expressed hurt, or blamed other people, we could get what we wanted and needed from them, particularly our parents. To survive, all of us learned that by making other people feel wrong, bad, guilty, or sorry for us, we could manipulate our world and thus receive the energy, love, attention, and support we needed at a given point in our growth and evolution. We didn't know any better.

But now we do. And once we're aware of this dynamic, we can never truly go back—especially if we want to master loving ourselves unconditionally or fulfill our life's purpose. Ultimately, in every moment of every day we're either unconsciously channeling our life force energy toward blaming other people and circumstances outside of ourselves or, we're consciously channeling our life force energy toward healing ourselves and creating the healthy, happy, and fulfilling life that we all desire. Thus, if we truly want to be free from our suffering, and also content both personally and professionally, we have no choice but to take one hundred percent responsibility for everything in our lives. This means we have to stop blaming other people, factors, and circumstances outside of ourselves for how we feel or for where we are in our lives, because our lives are, and will always be, completely our own creations.

Even in situations where we've experienced abuse, whether physical, sexual, or verbal, it's crucial that we eventually 'find the light' by looking for the purpose or lesson that the trauma or pain served. In certain circumstances this can indeed be extremely difficult, however, at some point we have to stop blaming others as well as ourselves so we can move forward and truly be happy. To achieve this we're called to rise above all forms of blame and to expand our perception on the meaning of our life experiences so we can finally stick up for, honor, and respect ourselves now in the ways we haven't always known how to. Thus, regardless of how powerless we may have felt in the past, we're all challenged to heal the pain and anger present within us now so we can exercise forgiveness and compassion for everyone involved and then move forward freely, empowered, and much more aware.

Like the old cliché – *if it doesn't kill you it only makes you stronger* – every life experience, regardless of how painful, scary, or seemingly "wrong" it was, actually introduces us to our inherent strength and unlimited capacity to overcome any obstacle we face. Both personally and professionally I've witnessed people who've endured the most extreme abuses imaginable reclaim their health and happiness by accepting their pain-filled wounds as necessary experiences that served them in fulfilling their life's larger purpose to bring unconditional love, compassion, forgiveness, and wisdom into our world.

No one saves us but ourselves. No one can and no
one may. We ourselves must walk the path.

—BUDDHA

At the deepest level of our being, we can never truly love and respect ourselves when we're blaming other people or external circumstances for any reason, because it's impossible to feel good about ourselves and our lives when we perceive ourselves to be a victim. When we blame, even in the smallest of ways, we unconsciously commit to remain trapped in the painful and miserable situations, relationships, memories, and self-destructive patterns that all of us, deep down, want freedom from. In essence, when we blame or play the victim we actually give our personal power, energy, and happiness away to whomever or whatever we're trying to project responsibility onto.

Having said that, we can only find healing, happiness, and self-respect to the degree we are willing to be accountable for our lives. To liberate our soul from suffering we must eventually acknowledge that our lives, as they manifest in the outside world, are just the product of our own beliefs, thoughts, emotions, actions, and spoken words. Our lives are ultimately just the accumulated result of all the beliefs we've ever believed, all the thoughts we've ever thought, all the emotions we've ever felt, all the actions we've ever taken, and all the words we've ever spoken in all of the past moments leading up to this moment.

Likewise, the life we experience from this moment onward is also entirely our own creation. The beliefs, thoughts, emotions, actions, and spoken words that are alive within us right now, and that we're expressing out into the world, are the energy and vibration with which we're both creating and attracting all of our coming life experiences. Thus, the only way to transform the pain-filled wounds that continue to surface in those moments, situations, and relationships in which we feel ourselves to be victims is to accept full responsibility for the parts of our lives we have unintentionally created. The more we choose to do this, the more we empower ourselves to redirect our life force energy here in the present toward healing our wounds, loving ourselves, and creating the joyful, liberating experience of life that we deserve.

I do not believe in a fate that falls on men however they act; but
I do believe in a fate that falls on them unless they act.

—BUDDHA

Ironically, the people we tend to blame or feel victimized around always represent the relationships in which we compromise, abandon, betray, and hurt ourselves in some way. Thus, once we finally realize how self-destructive it is when we do not love, honor, value, and express ourselves in every situation, we can finally take responsibility for our own health and happiness by choosing, moment after moment, to clarify, focus on, and do what we truly want to and need to for ourselves without fear.

At some point our wise inner voice declares, "I do not want to suffer anymore or give away my personal power, health, and happiness to anyone or anything." And it's in these moments that we finally choose not to waste our time or energy on reactively blaming other people or feeling sorry for ourselves. Rather, we choose to break through our victim-filled and blame-filled manipulations to get clear about what we love, want, and need here in the present moment so we can move forward in creating it consciously.

The more deeply we love ourselves, the faster we reclaim our vital life force energy, health, and happiness from the people and circumstances that we blame or play the victim with whenever we're aware that we're sabotaging ourselves in this way. Once we respect ourselves enough to stop hurting ourselves and thus accept one hundred percent responsibility for everything within us and within our lives, both from the past and in the present, we're immediately empowered to create each day in a way where we're truly at peace, purpose-driven, and fulfilled.

As we master this process as it unfolds in every moment, situation, and relationship, we finally, and thankfully, begin to enjoy life as much as possible each day. When we stop blaming external forces for the life we've created and take responsibility for everything that we believe, think, feel, do, and say, in every moment of every day, we're (1) naturally freed from our suffering and (2) granted access to the infinite source of all that we seek that's just waiting in the depths of our very own being.

Heal Yourself Now Questions

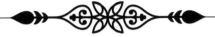

In which situations and relationships do you
feel yourself to be a victim right now?

Where and with whom in the past have
you felt yourself to be a victim?

Whom and what do you blame for where you are in life right
now or for what you're doing in your life right now?

Whom do you still give your personal power,
health, and happiness away to?

Whom and what do you constantly complain about? What can
you do to change your approach to the situation or person?

Do you still blame your parents, your partner, your spouse,
your children, God, or anyone else for any reason?

Whom do you expect to save you, rescue you,
take care of you, or make you happy?

Whom do you try to save, rescue, take care of, or make happy?

If you've ever experienced physical or sexual abuse, either as a
child or adult, can you see how the trauma may have taught you
the importance of (1) sticking up for yourself, (2) expressing
yourself, (3) forgiving yourself, and (4) forgiving others?

Once again, where and with whom in your life are you
compromising yourself and your inner truth?

What can you focus your energy on today that represents
you loving and valuing yourself and therefore honoring
what you love to do, want to do, or need to do?

Love Yourself Now Affirmations

I am not a victim. I never have been and I never will be.

I am one hundred percent responsible for my
life and for everything I experience.

I am one hundred percent responsible for the life I have created.

I am one hundred percent responsible for the
life I experience from today onward.

I will not blame anyone or anything ever
again. I will not give my power away.

I don't need to get sick to be loved, appreciated, or recognized.

I have everything I need within me to
create a fulfilling life that I love.

I cannot save or rescue anyone. They must heal and fulfill themselves.

No one can save me or rescue me. I must heal and fulfill myself.

I am ready to stop blaming myself. It's ok to
move on, forgive, and be happy.

I chose everything in my life in order to fulfill my
life's purpose and realize my greatest potential.

CHAPTER EIGHT

Love and Heal Your Inner Child

In every real man a child is hidden that wants to play.

—FRIEDRICH NIETZSCHE

> *Wherever you are, please take a few slow, deep breaths into your belly. Please also feel your whole body, from your feet all the way up to the crown of your head, and then down to your fingertips. Please surrender fully and accept everything that you're thinking, feeling, and experiencing here in this moment. Please be present to your body and your breath.*

The term "wounded inner child" typically refers to the emotional pain experienced during childhood that currently remains unhealed within us. The reason why it's optimal to address this topic at this stage in the book is because our psychological and emotional wounds from childhood are directly connected to the situations and relationships that are currently full of victimhood and blame.

In order to love and heal ourselves fully, we subconsciously create experiences in the present that mirror experiences from our past, often from childhood, so we can (1) transform the associated pain that is still stored within us and (2) learn the important soul lessons necessary to fulfill our life's purpose and awaken spiritually. In other words, if we have not fully healed a past experience or period that was painful or confusing, then we will instinctually create situations in the present that reflect back to us the unresolved emotions from the original incident(s), ultimately so we can make peace with our past, love ourselves more deeply, and move forward.

The feelings of hurt and powerlessness that always co-arise with our patterns of blame and victimhood actually exist so we may bring unconditional love and awareness to the child within us and heal these deeply rooted wounds from the past. Through giving ourselves the unconditional love that most of us did not receive as children, we can, in a sense, become the enlightened parents we never had and thus recreate our childhood. By using our innate intelligence to revisit past memories and experiences that were painful, scary, traumatic, or love-deprived, we can fill these dark inner spaces with the love, compassion, and belief in ourselves that we've always needed.

Psychoanalysis is in essence a cure through love.

—Sigmund Freud

Another way of looking at the process of healing our wounded inner child focuses primarily on the subtle relationship between our body and our soul. Although our physical body and our soul are not actually separate in any way, from this particular perspective, when we encounter painful, scary, or traumatic experiences as children, parts of us, or fragments of our soul, actually disassociate and leave our body until we feel it's safe to return. In these instances, the psychological and emotional pain is often too overwhelming for us to feel and process, so we repress both the emotion and the memory into some part of our physical body. This process literally pushes fragments of our soul out into the space surrounding our physical body (typically called our energy body). In other words, the overwhelming emotional pain often felt during childhood becomes bottled up in a way where it fills both the open spaces and the cells that make up our physical body, thereby forcing parts of our soul outside our body until we're ready to heal these emotional wounds and thus embody these parts of our soul fully once again.

Knowing this, we all can heal our early emotional pain through creating a loving and safe environment within ourselves and our lives now. More specifically, we can go back both in time and in memory and then invite all of ourselves, or all of our soul, back into our body by bringing the wisdom of our lived experience to our inner child. One of the best ways to achieve this is to open a dialogue between ourselves now and ourselves as a child, and the practices found at the end of this chapter will guide you through this process.

As you move forward, please keep in mind that healing our wounded inner child is a process that varies for each person. For some of us, this lifetime has been full of abuse and trauma, thus it will take a little longer to re-integrate all of our soul back into our body and our life. For others, this life has not been quite as traumatic, so the process of re-integrating all of our soul will not be as intensive. Either way, our innate intelligence already knows the best and most natural approach to our unique healing and personal awakening.

Even if our childhood was extremely traumatic or painful, through giving ourselves the love we have always deserved, we can still liberate ourselves from our suffering and reawaken to life's ever-present beauty. Eventually, through caring for our inner child, the evolutionary force of the universe will awaken the light and the love within every cell of our body and every situation in our life, because life was always meant to be a wonderful experience.

Overall, our lives as human beings can be viewed simply as the journey from healing our wounded inner child to embodying an enlightened form of our inner child, because as we heal our repressed emotional pain and master the lessons we came here to learn, we not only rediscover the innocence, purity, openness, and vulnerability of a child, but we also exemplify true wisdom, love, intelligence, and self-awareness. Thus, the more loving attention we direct inward toward healing our inner child, the sooner we welcome home the parts of ourselves that we've lost touch with and the more joyful and simple our lives become.

Writing a Letter *to* Your Inner Child

Step 1.

Please find a quiet place where you feel
safe to be open and vulnerable.

Step 2.

Please imagine yourself in the most beautiful place on earth. What
is the most beautiful place to you? Where is it? What does it feel like
to be there? Please visualize it, feel into it, and connect to this place.

Step 3.

Please imagine yourself sitting somewhere in this beautiful place,
and please imagine that your five-year-old self has now come to sit
with you. Then, connecting to yourself at five years of age, please
ask yourself as the adult what you would tell your younger self if
given the chance. What did he or she need to know or hear at this
age but was never told? If you could go back in time and encourage
or affirm anything to your five-year-old self, what would you say?

Step 4.

After taking some time to contemplate the questions above,
please write a letter to your five-year-old self. Please begin
with "Dear [your name]," and please express everything that
you would say to yourself as a five-year-old child if given the
opportunity. Then, please take a few slow, deep breaths and
allow yourself to fully feel and experience whatever is true for
you. Please notice any memories that arise from the past.

Step 5.

Please repeat steps three and four while connecting with your ten-year-old self, your fifteen-year-old self, and your twenty-year-old self. Please feel free to do this with any additional age(s) that you feel inspired to do so with.

Writing a Letter *from* Your Inner Child

Step 1.

Please find a quiet place where you feel
safe to be open and vulnerable.

Step 2.

Please imagine yourself in the most beautiful place on earth. What
is the most beautiful place to you? Where is it? What does it feel like
to be there? Please visualize it, feel into it, and connect to this place.

Step 3.

Please imagine yourself sitting somewhere in this beautiful place,
and please imagine that your five-year-old self has now come to
sit with you. Then, connecting to yourself at five years of age,
please ask your five-year-old self what he or she wants to tell
you as the adult. What does he or she want you to know or hear
right now in your life? What wisdom and healing does your five-
year-old self need to encourage in you as an adult right now?

Step 4.

After taking some time to contemplate the questions above, please
write a letter from your five-year-old self addressed to your adult
self. Please begin with "Dear [your name]," and please express
everything that your five-year-old self wants you, the adult, to
know, hear, and remember. Then, please take a few slow, deep
breaths and allow yourself to fully feel and experience whatever
is true for you. Please notice any situations or relationships
that you're being guided to address in your life right now.

Love Yourself Now Affirmations

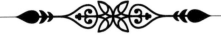

I forgive myself for choosing the parents I chose.

I am grateful for the important life lessons I learned in my childhood.

I forgive myself for not sticking up for myself in the past.

I forgive myself for compromising and abandoning myself for love.

I am willing to forgive anyone who hurt, abused, or mistreated me.

I forgive myself for any abuse or pain that I did
not know how to protect myself from.

I forgive myself and others for any abuse or pain that I witnessed.

It was not my fault. I am not to blame.

I am smart, capable, attractive, loveable,
respectable, and secure in myself.

I am not a child anymore. I will not allow
my past to punish me any longer.

I was born to enjoy a wonderful and magical life.

I was born to have fun, to grow, to learn, to explore, and to love.

I came into this world to create joy and beauty.

Little [your name], I love you.

It's okay for me to have fun and joy in my life!

Adults need toys too!

Additional Practice for Healing Your Inner Child

When you have some space, I recommend finding a picture, or pictures, of yourself as a child. Then, I recommend looking at the "little you" in these pictures and expressing some of the affirmations listed above. For example, look at your younger self and say, "[Your name], I love you. You deserve to be loved just as you are. You are enough." Please try this with as many photos as you'd like. This can be a very healing and liberating exercise if you allow it to be.

CHAPTER NINE

Break Free of Your Ego

There is a kind of experience so different from anything the ego can offer that you will never want to cover or hide it again. … The ego is afraid of the spirit's joy, because once you have experienced it you will withdraw all protection from the ego, and become totally without investment in fear.

—*A Course in Miracles*

Wherever you are, please take a few slow, deep breaths into your belly. Please also feel your whole body, from your feet all the way up to the crown of your head, and then down to your fingertips. Please surrender fully and accept everything that you're thinking, feeling, and experiencing here in this moment. Please be present to your body and your breath.

O ur ego is not our enemy. Contrary to what most of us believe, we all create the cocoon of our ego as an act of unconditional self-love to protect us until we're ready to fully embody our soul's true nature. The primary function of our ego is to protect our soul in the same way the cocoon protects the caterpillar throughout its metamorphosis into a butterfly. Our ego acts as our guardian until we're ready to break through our fears and live as a free and full expression of who and what we truly are each and every day.

The development of our ego is a natural part of our soul's growth and evolution. In the same way the caterpillar must create a cocoon to protect itself throughout its transformation into a butterfly, we too must develop the cocoon of our ego to protect us throughout our own process of transformation, healing, and awakening. The caterpillar is the creator of its cocoon, but it is not the cocoon itself. Similarly, we are the creator of our ego, but we are not the ego itself. Without the cocoon the caterpillar could never become a butterfly, and without the ego we could never embody a free and full expression of our inherent brilliance.

With this in mind, through loving ourselves unconditionally in the present moment we can (1) heal the psychological, emotional, and physical pain that our ego exists to protect us from feeling and (2) create our most liberated and joyful life. If we truly want to experience the inner freedom and happiness that we all desire, each of us is called to open both our heart and our mind to the larger reality beyond the cold comfort our soul's protective cocoon.

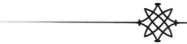

To break free from the limitations of our ego as soon as possible, it's important to remember how and why we created this defensive aspect of our personality in the first place.

As we've touched on before, the world didn't always feel very safe growing up, so we all intuitively created a protective shell through which we could relate to both ourselves and to life. The overwhelming emotional and psychic energies that bombarded us as children were often too much for us to feel, process, and understand on our own, and this drove all of us to develop the cocoon of our ego to protect us from the painful and confusing energies that we encountered on a daily basis.

In our desire to individuate from the world around us each of us organically closed ourselves off and separated ourselves from the outside world because instinctually we felt that doing so would give us some control over what was occurring in our lives. Out of an inherent love for ourselves, each of us built an all-encompassing psycho-energetic cocoon of perceived safety and security to protect our hearts, knowing that one day we would finally cultivate the necessary awareness and skills to honor our emotions on our own and thus liberate ourselves.

Since a very large number of us did not have people in our lives who had cultivated the awareness to lovingly mirror back to us what we were feeling as children, we never learned how to consciously identify or express the thoughts and emotions that we were experiencing. Instead, many of us learned to reject, repress, deny, avoid, and hide what we felt and thought in order to (1) survive and (2) have our needs met to some degree. And this developing internal relationship between ourselves and our world gave birth to the defensive aspects of our personality.

The degree to which our ego initially developed depended upon the amount of protection we intuitively felt we needed as children. Thus the strength and thickness of this protective layer of our personality varies for each of us depending on how painful and confusing our lives have been. If the family and larger environments that we grew up in did not support us to lovingly honor, process, and be present to what we felt on a daily basis (and most did not), we would've built up a much stronger ego and disconnected from our emotions to a larger degree because we didn't know how to lovingly process, understand, and attend to our feelings for ourselves. If, on the other hand, we grew up with emotionally aware and present parents, then we would have been supported in understanding, processing, and expressing our emotions and would not have needed to build up such a strong or large protective shell.

As we "mature," most of us just remain trapped in our protective cocoon—especially those of us with big egos—because we never learn how to lovingly attend to or heal our unresolved emotional pain. The safe and familiar confines of our ego often become comfortable, simply because we fear facing the painful emotions that live beneath the surface of our conscious awareness. If we don't wake up and reconnect with our deep inner truths by the time we reach all the responsibilities of "adulthood," most of us just continue living our lives disconnected from our soul and completely identify with our ego. In fact, an alarmingly large number of us end up settling for a limited existence, because liberating ourselves would entail feeling all of the love as well as all of the fear that we've denied for so long. To the majority of us, it simply appears easier to continue living in cold comfort, hiding out in the familiarity of our protected world. Having lived with our hearts closed to our own inner magnificence for so long, we've mistakenly come to identify with the limiting voice of our ego rather than the expansive soul that's just waiting to break free.

Enter by the narrow gate; for wide is the gate and broad is the way that leads to destruction, and there are many who go in by it. Because narrow is the gate and difficult is the way which leads to life, and there are few who find it.

—MATTHEW 7:13–14

In trying to protect us our ego keeps us reacting to life, constantly running from ourselves here in the present moment. In fact, the thoughts that just don't stop coming are merely symptoms of undigested emotions and experiences that are currently being guarded by our ego. This protective aspect of our personality very skillfully avoids whatever is true internally and externally by constantly manufacturing thoughts about the past and the future to prevent us from feeling the hurt and confusion that remain alive within us here and now.

As a result of this dynamic, many of us remain trapped in our head, stuck reacting to life in ways that stop us from finding the inner peace, health, happiness, and fulfillment we desire. We're not aware of it but in constantly denying our psychological, emotional, and physical pain, we not only create more sickness and misery, we also cover up the abundant source of love within us that is intended to heal, fulfill, and sustain each of us.

Ultimately, when we fail to transform the pain and confusion that we've disconnected from and shoved away over the years, we start compounding the suffering that we were initially trying to avoid. In this way, our ego's purposeful protection, which is necessary to a point, eventually begins to create additional pain on top of the suffering it was originally created to shelter us from. Thus, in constantly disconnecting from or numbing ourselves to our inner struggles, we not only avoid healing them, but we also avoid understanding their root cause.

An analogy that demonstrates the purpose and function of our ego quite well is that of using painkillers to relieve physical pain. In the same way we might take a painkiller to relieve ourselves from feeling the pain of, say, a headache, our egos relieve us from feeling pain that is hard for us to handle at particular points in time. In taking a painkiller to remedy a headache, the underlying conditions that caused the headache are still present; we've just numbed ourselves to them. We experience temporary relief and believe that our pain has gone away, but in reality the pain and its source actually remain unhealed.

Our ego's protective function is similar to that of a painkiller's function in relieving the pain of a headache. Our ego temporarily disconnects us from our pain so we can function and carry on in our lives. Just like a painkiller, the relief our ego brings is only temporary in nature, because the pain and its source still remain unhealed. Furthermore, the same pain that was temporarily masked will surface again and again until we understand its underlying cause, heal it, and therefore liberate ourselves from it for good.

From this perspective, if we have chronic headaches and we continue taking painkillers on a regular basis without looking deeper into the source of the pain, besides developing an immunity to the painkilling function and thus needing higher doses, we'll also begin building up toxicity in our bodies from all the chemicals contained within the painkillers. In situations like this, we live unaware of our affliction's root cause and the affliction itself remains unhealed. Our approach to managing our pain, which once seemed supportive and loving, unfortunately just becomes a further source of suffering.

Once again, the same can also be said for our ego. We all unconsciously create our ego in order to protect us from feeling pain. But eventually we create additional suffering for ourselves because in continuously disconnecting from our pain, we not only avoid healing it; we also avoid addressing its source. Thus, our initial way of managing our psychological and emotional pain, which once provided temporary and effective relief, just creates more misery and sickness in our lives when we do not transform the underlying issues.

For most of us it's not until our suffering becomes so intense and compounded that our protective shell cracks and we open to approaching ourselves and our lives from new perspectives. Most of us tend to be so stubborn and closed-minded that life has to get so difficult before we'll finally surrender and change the ways that we relate to ourselves and our world. Quite often it's not until we're somehow forced to face our fears that we finally open our heart fully to feeling our way through life and thus break free from the protective aspects of our personality that we're all destined to outgrow.

Whether the catalyst is an intimate relationship, the death of a loved one, a suicidal depression, a newborn child, or an important goal or dream, the point always comes in our healing and spiritual growth where our ego becomes limiting and unhealthy. When this time inevitably arrives, we're all blessed with an opportunity to love ourselves and release our unconscious need for protection, control, and separation.

The creation of our ego is indeed a necessary and purposeful part of our soul's evolutionary unfolding, because we must create what we perceive to be a separate self in order to fulfill our life's purpose and master loving ourselves unconditionally. All of us must unconsciously love and protect ourselves until we're ready to consciously and lovingly liberate ourselves from all of our self-imposed limitations. However, just as the creation of our ego is a necessary step in mastering an unconditional love for ourselves, so too is our eventual liberation from it. As we grow in both awareness and love for ourselves we're naturally guided from within to break through our fear-based defense mechanisms so we can heal all of the uncomfortable emotions that we've repressed throughout our lives. Thankfully, once we're prepared to face our suffering directly, life itself does everything in its power to support us in breaking free from our inner limitations, ultimately so the inner peace, health, happiness, and fulfillment that we're looking for may finally surface from deep within our being.

CHAPTER TEN

Remember Who You Are and Why You Came Here

When I was five years old, my mother always told me that happiness was the key to life. When I went to school, they asked me what I wanted to be when I grew up. I wrote down "happy." They told me I didn't understand the assignment, and I told them they didn't understand life.

—JOHN LENNON

> *Wherever you are, please take a few slow, deep breaths into your belly. Please also feel your whole body, from your feet all the way up to the crown of your head, and then down to your fingertips. Please surrender fully and accept everything that you're thinking, feeling, and experiencing here in this moment. Please be present to your body and your breath.*

The questions "Who am I?" and "Why am I here?" are at the heart of every human life. Thus, to free ourselves from our suffering and master loving ourselves unconditionally, we're all called to remember, with crystal clarity, who we truly are and why we're really here. Above all else, understanding that your life has a purpose and that all life is purposeful is the one thing that will guide you, empower you, and inspire you to persist on your healing and spiritual journey toward complete self-mastery and self-realization.

Like the destiny of every human being, your destiny entails mastering unconditional self-love so you may embody the love that you are, and in so doing find complete psychological, emotional, physical, financial, and spiritual freedom in your daily life. In other words, through loving yourself unconditionally in every moment, situation, and relationship, you cannot help but fulfill your life's purpose to create a healthy, happy, and prosperous life that is in harmony with all that exists.

Believe it or not, each of us is destined to awaken to the God-nature of our soul and thereby reach spiritual enlightenment in this lifetime. Therefore, just like all human beings, your destiny is to realize your own greatest potential and to live your life abundantly, to the fullest, while consciously transforming any perceived obstacle to experiencing life in this way.

Whether or not you choose to align with this ultimate purpose is entirely up to you, but the fact remains that you and I are here to break through every self-imposed limitation, negative belief, and form of suffering to embody a unique, free, and full expression of who and what we truly are.

Knowing this, our intentions, choices, and actions in each and every moment are either leading us closer to fulfilling our life's purpose and therefore to loving ourselves unconditionally or, they are creating more pain, misery, and sickness in our lives. In fact, every experience that we've had since our conception right up until this very moment has been teaching us to lovingly accept, forgive, honor, value, respect, express, trust in, stick up for, and believe in ourselves so we may heal our suffering completely and thereby rediscover the clarity and bliss that are inherent to our soul's true nature.

> *I searched for God, and found only myself. I*
> *searched for myself, and found only God.*

> —SUFI PROVERB

From an elevated perspective, a very large part of our purpose in life involves remembering that what we tend to call our "self," our "soul," or our "spirit" is actually God manifesting in a unique form through what we perceive as our physical and nonphysical being. In other words, each one of us is a unique expression of God in human form. You and I, as well as every other person alive—regardless of skin color, religious belief, economic status, and cultural background—are irreplaceable manifestations of the intelligent and aware universe unfolding in the form of a human being.

In accepting this blasphemous truth we find our greatest liberation, because when we consciously own our unity with both God and the universe we realize that there's no point in blaming anyone or anything outside of ourselves for how we feel or for the lives we've created. More importantly, through recognizing this ultimate reality, we finally empower ourselves to heal our suffering completely, because in accepting total responsibility, we stop giving our health and happiness away to people and circumstances outside ourselves and thus reclaim the energy necessary to heal our lives and fulfill the purpose for which we were born.

The true or primary purpose of your life cannot be found on the outer level. It does not concern what you do but what you are—that is to say, your state of consciousness ... Your inner purpose is to awaken ... It is that simple. You share that purpose with every other person on the planet- because it is the purpose of humanity. Your inner purpose is an essential part of the purpose of the whole, the universe and its emerging intelligence ... Finding and living in alignment with the inner purpose is the foundation for fulfilling your outer purpose. It is the basis for true success. Without that alignment, you can still achieve certain things through effort, struggle, determination, and sheer hard work or cunning. But there is no joy in such endeavor, and it invariably ends in some form of suffering.

—ECKHART TOLLE

Even though all of us begin our healing and spiritual journey by looking outside of ourselves for who we are as well as for the purpose of our lives, eventually we realize that no external person, situation, or relationship can truly give us the answers we're looking for. There will always come a time where we're forced to accept that it's only through looking within ourselves, through following the subtle whispers of our own heart and soul, and through trusting and believing in our own innate intelligence that we can find the love, clarity, passion, and joy we're all seeking.

The universal intelligence that expresses in, as, and through each of us is always guiding us forward toward our healthiest, happiest, and most fulfilling life. So once we're wholeheartedly committed to loving ourselves unconditionally we can surrender into the natural force and flow of life itself, which then leads us directly, and as effortlessly as possible, toward everything that we truly want and need.

Fulfilling our life's purpose to embody the enlightened and loving God-nature of our soul can only happen through focusing our attention inwardly on loving ourselves unconditionally day in and day out. In other words, we are called to value ourselves enough to follow our heart and go after what we truly want and love, because when we do, we cannot help but find the freedom, joy, and peace that result from simply being ourselves and from doing what we were born to do.

> *Your work is to discover your work and then with*
> *all your heart to give yourself to it.*

> —BUDDHA

Most of us didn't learn this growing up but we are all destined to find our own unique place in the grand orchestra of human life. We're all meant to remember the intentional role we were born to play as an integral part of the one human family. To free ourselves from our suffering, therefore, we must both understand and accept that we're all pioneers in our own lives. No one has ever, can ever, or will ever walk in our shoes, because we're all truly one of a kind.

Our unique path through life is ultimately uncharted territory, which means our personal destiny and awakening are unfolding in a way that is particular to our own karma, purpose, and inner evolution.

Thus, in each moment and with each breath we're all actually charting our own distinct course toward bringing the love that we are fully into this world.

As we go through the inner healing, strengthening, and awakening necessary to master relating to ourselves with unconditional love in every moment, situation, and relationship, the unique gifts and talents that we were born to share organically surface in the memory of our body, heart, and mind, essentially so we may create our lives based upon these deeply liberating inner truths. Thus, on a very personal level, beyond knowing the importance of creating a healthy relationship with yourself that is based on unconditional love, kindness, respect, and compassion, *no one can tell you exactly how* to go about fulfilling your life's purpose. We all have to (1) love ourselves daily, (2) listen to the subtle inner voice of our heart and soul, and (3) learn to follow this guidance into and through our deepest fears, doubts, and insecurities.

> *At the center of your being you have the answer; you know who you are and you know what you want.*

—LAO TZU

As we follow the inspirations of our heart more consistently, our choices and actions become driven less by external motivations or conditioning and more by the inner call of our soul, which is always guiding us forward toward our destiny and greatest potential. By honoring and valuing these inner truths in every moment, situation, and relationship, we naturally just come to know, without doubt or confusion, who we truly are and why we're really here.

Once we open our heart enough to remember that only love matters and that only love is real we organically let go of the aspects of ourselves and our lives that are not grounded in truth or love, because we know they do not support our health, happiness, or capacity to give back to life. Eventually we come to see so clearly that all of our life experiences, needs, desires, and dreams are simply lessons that were created to support us in fulfilling our life's purpose to love ourselves, others, and all life wholeheartedly. Finally, we realize that we simply were not born to suffer. Rather, we were born to enjoy living this beautiful life to the fullest alongside all our human brothers and sisters.

Heal Yourself Now Questions

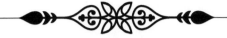

Are you happy and satisfied with the work you do on a daily basis?

If not, why not?

If you could do something that you love and are
passionate about each day and also support yourself
financially doing it, what would you choose to do?

Whom or what are you allowing to stop you from focusing on your
passions each day? What fears are holding you back? Are material
comfort and money more important than your health and happiness?

Who and what do you believe yourself to be? A body?
A soul? A spirit? The voice in your head?

Why are you here on earth? No one is here by accident,
so what gifts were you born to give to the world?

Can you remember what you dreamed of doing and being as a child?
Can you recall your sacred mission or soul contract in this lifetime?

Are you waiting for your children to age, your parents
to die, or your intimate relationship to end before you
start honoring your true needs and desires?

If so, why?

If you only had one year to live, what would you change?
What would you go do, experience, or accomplish?
Whom would you forgive? Whom would you reach out
to? Whom would you express yourself to fully?

Love Yourself Now Affirmations

I deserve to be happy.

I deserve to enjoy my life and my work each and every day.

I am destined to create a fulfilling life that I love.

I have everything I need to fulfill my life's
purpose and liberate my soul.

I am God in human form. I am pure, unconditional love.

I am exactly where I need to be to master loving myself.

I was not born to suffer. I am here to love, and to enjoy my life.

CHAPTER ELEVEN

Come Home to Life in the Present Moment

One must learn to love oneself with a wholesome and healthy love,
so that one can bear to be with oneself and need not roam.

—FRIEDRICH NIETZSCHE

> *Wherever you are, please take a few slow, deep breaths into your belly. Please also feel your whole body, from your feet all the way up to the crown of your head, and then down to your fingertips. Please surrender fully and accept everything that you're thinking, feeling, and experiencing here in this moment. Please be present to your body and your breath.*

Deep down we all want to feel "welcome," that we "belong," and that we are accepted unconditionally just the way we are. Ultimately we all just want to feel at home within ourselves and our lives. When we feel safe and secure to be ourselves, that no one is judging us, and that we can let our guard down and be vulnerable, our hearts open, naturally allowing the peace, joy, and love that are inherent to who we are to flow freely within us and then out into our lives. To feel the warm embrace of unconditional love that most of us associate with the idea of "home" is how we as human beings truly come to blossom and thrive in life. Even if our own experiences at "home," either as children or as adults, have never truly been as loving or as warm as we've wanted them to be, deep down we all know it's possible to live in and create supportive environments for ourselves that are full of kindness, respect, acceptance, compassion, and joy.

For various reasons, however, many of us still have not found, or created, the home that we're looking for. What we're rarely taught, and often don't realize, is that the one true home that we're all intuitively pursuing already exists within us just below the inner battles we're subconsciously doing everything in our power to avoid.

The only reason why any of us do not feel at home within ourselves and therefore within our lives here in the present moment is simply because we're reacting to and trying to escape the psychological, emotional, or physical pain that still remains unhealed within us. More specifically, most of us are currently running from life itself in the here and now, because we fear facing the aspects of ourselves, our lives, and our past that we have not fully welcomed, accepted, forgiven, honored, or learned to love unconditionally yet.

Thus, regardless of what coming home, going home, or being at home means to each of us as unique individuals, the home we're all looking for can never truly be found outside of ourselves. We can create loving and warm environments in the outer world, but doing so is always dependent on, and reflective of, how loving and warm we feel within and toward ourselves.

Sometimes we may think we've found our home in the outer world, maybe in another person or a specific place, but if we do not wholeheartedly love, value, and accept ourselves, then eventually the fact that we are not at home within ourselves will always resurface to be addressed. This is why coming home to life in the present moment, moment after moment, day after day, is one of the most important keys to (1) loving ourselves unconditionally and (2) transforming all of our suffering.

Although we may think there was, or will be, a more opportune time, we cannot love ourselves or liberate our soul in some long-gone past or in some distant fantasy of the future. We can only love and therefore heal, fulfill, and free ourselves right here in this very moment by creating a loving, safe environment within our own body, heart, and mind—starting now.

The secret of health for both mind and body is not to mourn
for the past, worry about the future, or anticipate troubles, but
to live in the present moment wisely and earnestly.

—BUDDHA

Through consistently living with our awareness focused on what is true in this moment, here and now, we empower ourselves to illuminate everything that must be transformed, healed, and loved within us to find lasting inner peace, health, happiness, and fulfillment in our lives. Over time, through consistently observing our inner reality in this way, we're able to identify the negative, aggressive, and self-destructive ways in which we currently relate to and talk to ourselves that are not grounded in love. By focusing our consciousness on these inner truths, we're then empowered to bring a loving presence deep into our body, heart, and mind and thereby transform whatever is blocking or sabotaging our natural health, wealth, and happiness.

Through relating to ourselves with the love, kindness, and compassion that we deserve we eventually realize that the psychological, emotional, physical, financial, and spiritual freedom we're seeking is already available right here in this very moment. In other words, besides liberating ourselves from the vicious cycles of feeling held back by the past or feeling worried about the future, through coming home to life in the present moment, we find that there's always been an ocean of unconditional love, peace, joy, and fulfillment within us beneath the anxiety, pain, unhappiness, and dissatisfaction that have resulted from our unhealthy, aggressive, and self-destructive inner relationship with ourselves.

Thus, the sole requirement in coming home to the limitless source of all that we seek within us is that we pay attention, as much as possible, to every breath that we take, every belief that we believe, every thought that we think, every emotion that we feel, every word that we speak, and every action that we take, and then simply allow the love that we are to radiate from every cell in our body and then infuse every moment, situation, and relationship in our lives.

> *If you will but turn to Me, and will carefully watch for and study these impressions which you are receiving every moment, and will learn to trust them, and thus to wait upon and rest in Me, putting all your faith in Me, verily I will guide you in all your ways; I will solve for you all your problems, make easy all your work, and you will be led among green pastures, beside the still waters of life.*

—*The Impersonal Life*

From a broader perspective, consistently focusing on the present moment is also our pathway home to God, to the unlimited creative force of the universe, who lives and has its being within and through our lives. In other words, this moment here and now is also where we remember and experience our oneness with the infinite, loving intelligence that created and sustains all life on our planet as well as all that exists throughout the entire universe.

Practically speaking, when we're present to life in the here and now, our inner wellspring of all-pervading awareness and wisdom expands from deep within us, providing us with the necessary insight to move forward in our personal growth and spiritual evolution. When we open our body, heart, and mind to the abundant, ever-present source of intelligence within us, we simultaneously open to the entire universal field of consciousness and energy that both permeates and fills everyone and everything that exists. This field that we're one with, but most often closed to, then comes pouring through our being, supporting us and illuminating exactly what we must transform, heal, and let go of in order to love ourselves unconditionally, fulfill our life's purpose, and realize our greatest potential.

Hence, the deeper our awareness runs into this very moment, into each breath of life itself, the more we can harness the infinite source of love, wisdom, and healing energy, which is always available both within us and all around us, and then channel it toward creating and achieving what we want and need most in life. Thankfully, underneath all of the thoughts, fears, and uncomfortable emotions that we react to and run from here in the present moment there is only peace, joy, and love within us. So when we're finally prepared to surrender to life in the here and now we naturally come home to rest and rejuvenate in these soul-nurturing and life-giving energies.

At the end of every spiritual discipline we find that this very moment exists eternally as the one and only gateway home to feeling and knowing the abundant wealth, magnificence, divinity, and wholeness that are inherent to our soul's true nature. The suffering, restlessness, unhappiness, and dis-ease that we experience are merely forms of homesickness guiding us back to an awareness of God and love within us.

Heal Yourself Now Questions

In this moment what are you feeling in your body,
your heart, and your mind? Do you feel tense, closed,
and anxious or relaxed, open, and at peace?

How is the quality of your breathing? Is it deep and slow or shallow
and fast? Can you breathe deeply and slowly into your lower belly
and lower back? Please try to and then notice what and how you feel.

Where in your body do you feel pain, tension, or discomfort?
Can you focus your awareness on that area and then
breathe deeply into it, allowing it to open and relax?

Do you believe that you are merely your thoughts and the
voice in your head? If so, then who and what is it inside
of you that can observe the thoughts and voices in your
head? Through focusing on your breath, can you feel the
space, peace, and stillness underneath your thoughts?

What does the word *home* mean to you? Do you feel at home within
yourself and also in your physical home? Did you feel at home in
your physical house growing up as a child? If not, why not?

Do you feel at home with the people you live with today? What
about the people you work with? If not, why not? If you're not
completely satisfied with your physical home, what does your ideal
living environment look like and feel like? Please describe it in as
much detail as possible and please do not limit yourself in any way.
If you're not completely satisfied with your work environment,
what does your ideal workspace look like and feel like? Once
again, please describe it in as much detail as possible and please do
not limit yourself in any way. (I highly recommend that you write
out your answers to this question, because doing so will help you
create ideal living and working environments as soon as possible.)

Love Yourself Now Affirmations

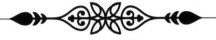

I deserve to feel good wherever I am.

My one true home is within my own heart and soul.

I am home. Welcome home, [your name].

I am worthy and deserving of a beautiful, loving home.

I am so much more than the voice in my head.

Underneath my thoughts I am free, peaceful, and full of love.

My physical pain and health concerns are
guiding me home to my true self.

My breath is my pathway home in every moment.

My suffering is asking me to fulfill my life's destined purpose.

CHAPTER TWELVE

Inhale Life Deeply
and Slowly

The mind can go in a thousand directions, but on this beautiful path, I walk in peace. With each step, the wind blows. With each step, a flower blooms…

Smile, breathe and go slowly.

—THICH NHAT HANH

> *Wherever you are, please take a few slow, deep breaths into your belly. Please also feel your whole body, from your feet all the way up to the crown of your head, and then down to your fingertips. Please surrender fully and accept everything that you're thinking, feeling, and experiencing here in this moment. Please be present to your body and your breath.*

If we can learn to be present to our breath in any given moment, we can find our way back to the peace, health, happiness, fulfillment, and freedom that are already alive within us. Ultimately, each inhalation offers a pathway down into the depths of our being, where unlimited space and stillness are always patiently waiting.

Our breath is like an anchor that has the power to keep us centered during the most turbulent of times. Regardless of how strong a thought or an emotion is in our moment-to-moment experience, we'll always find a wealth of joy, clarity, and love deep within us. Through our breath we can immediately step out of the illusory past and future into the truth of life in the here and now, where happiness and peace are eternally present no matter what's occurring. Thus, if we can intentionally practice dropping our awareness out of our heads by following our breath deep into our bodies, we can find acceptance, harmony, and courage in any moment or situation.

The primary reason why most of us typically breathe at very shallow depths, specifically into our throat and upper chest, is because we've repressed and stored so many uncomfortable emotions deep within our body that we ultimately fear feeling. However, through consciously focusing our attention on breathing slowly, deeply, and fully, specifically into our belly and then into our lungs, we allow the energy that's become trapped in our head as confusion and obsessive thinking, as well as the energy that's become trapped in our heart as anxiety and stress, to literally melt and drop, and then fill our body in a balanced and harmonious way.

To truly find the space, peace, and stillness that exist deep within us, we must eventually make the challenging but necessary journey from our head down through our heart, and into the very deepest parts of our being. At some point in our quest for lasting health, happiness, and fulfillment, we must find the courage to feel all of the hurt, anxiety, anger, insecurity, fear, guilt, and shame that we've shoved so deeply into the cells, organs, and spaces that make up our physical body.

Ultimately, the more deeply we breathe, the more deeply we feel, and it's only through feeling life deeply and fully that we can truly heal our bodies, hearts, and minds completely. In fact, there is a direct correlation between the fullness of our breath and the fullness of our lives, because we can only live our lives as fully as we're prepared to inhale the life force itself. Thus the more fully we inhale the life-giving energy of oxygenated breath, the more we actually enjoy being alive each day.

If you correct your mind, the rest of your life will fall into place.

—LAO TZU

As we've explored in previous chapters, a large number of us are not truly at peace, happy, or satisfied in our lives. However, on a deeper level, most of us are literally and physically not at peace, happy, or satisfied being in our bodies. The main reason why any of us would not find it enjoyable both within our body and our life is solely because of the uncomfortable emotions that we've created, repressed, and stored within our being.

This particular dynamic is one of the largest obstacles we must overcome on our way home to the source of peace, health, happiness, fulfillment, and unconditional love deep within us. In every moment that we do not inhale deeply and fully, we not only allow our old emotional wounds to fester and become toxic, but we also allow ourselves to pile additional pain on top of the already stagnant discomfort that we've unintentionally created and left unresolved. When we look at the process of breathing in this light, it becomes clear that each moment actually offers us an opportunity to love ourselves, heal ourselves, and fulfill ourselves by making a conscious choice to focus on inhaling the breath of life as deeply and as fully as we can.

We all know that human life would not be possible without oxygen, so if there's one thing that holds the power to give us more life and vitality than any other factor in our experience, our breath is by far the one. With this in mind, through intentionally breathing into every space inside our belly, back, chest, and shoulders, we can fill these areas with the life-giving and life-healing energies that are infinitely available, everywhere, all of the time.

Furthermore, through focusing our attention on inhaling as deeply and as slowly as we can, we simultaneously allow our awareness to expand beyond our head so it may fill every cell and corner of our being. The natural byproduct of this process is a deep, tangible, understanding of our unity with the ocean of energy and oxygen that fills all of the spaces and environments around us. Hence, simply through breathing in life as wholeheartedly as we're able to, we begin to remember that we're not separate from anyone or anything that exists. Through mindful, deep breathing we eventually reawaken to our oneness with both the universe and with all life, and we also rediscover the infinite potential energy and life-giving force that exists in every particle, atom, and molecule that surrounds us and gives form to our being.

Once you realize that the road is the goal, and that you are always on the road, not to reach a goal but to enjoy its beauty and its wisdom, life ceases to be a task and becomes natural and simple. In itself an ecstasy.

—NISARGADATTA MAHARAJ

All of us tend to make life much more complicated and difficult than it needs to be, mainly because we reject and deny so much of what we think and feel. In fact, as we've already seen, it's this pattern over time that creates all of the stress, struggle, and sickness that we experience in our lives. Having said that, I believe I'm not alone in expressing that life has felt quite hard at times. I also believe I'm not alone in saying that I often hear other people talk about how difficult life is, or has been, for them as well.

Through my own intensive healing and spiritual journey, as well as through my professional work with a large variety of people, I've come to realize that life itself is not actually hard; we just feel it to be so quite regularly because we never learned to fully face, feel, and heal the uncomfortable emotions that come with being human. Consequently, this emotional pain that we do everything in our power to protect ourselves from feeling just continues to build up over time, making life *feel* much harder than it needs to be.

For those of us who grew up feeling unloved, misunderstood, or unsupported, life can indeed feel challenging while we're learning to love, honor, value, and support ourselves. Thankfully, however, life actually becomes significantly easier when we stop resisting the flow of energy and emotion as it pulses throughout our being here in the present moment. In fact, once we learn to surrender fully to whatever we're thinking, feeling, or experiencing, we naturally release our inner fight and accept whatever is occurring both within us and around us without struggling at all.

It could be said that the single most important key to aligning ourselves with the harmonious flow of life itself is to master inhaling life deeply and slowly, because through intentionally cultivating this practice daily we can accept life as it is and allow life to unfold organically and enjoyably through our every thought, emotion, and experience.

Personally, I have found that underneath all of my thoughts and emotions there is an ever-present source of peace, stillness, and vital energy, and through consciously choosing to follow my breath deep into my body, I can find my way back to the inner freedom and happiness that I desire in any moment or situation. I have also found that, above all else, it is through breathing mindfully that we awaken to our oneness with the totality of life.

As we welcome our experiences fully through our breath in each moment, we become one with our experience and thus quite effortlessly put an end to our suffering. Simply by accepting our unity with all that exists here in the present moment, the pain we once felt from feeling isolated, insecure, mistreated, or unloved eventually just melts away into the loving silence from which it came, and all we're left with are the joy and bliss of our liberation.

Simple Deep-Breathing Meditation Practice

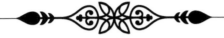

One of the most effective ways to cultivate effortlessness, ease, and total acceptance of life in each moment, situation, and relationship is through the following practice.

1. Gently place your tongue on the roof of your mouth. This connects two major energy channels/meridians in the body (used in traditional Chinese/Oriental medicine), which, once linked, create a harmonious, balanced, and continuous flow of energy throughout the body.

2. Then, with your eyes either open or closed, depending on where you are and what you're doing, please inhale slowly, deeply, and fully through your nose with the intention of filling your belly and lower back first and then your chest, your upper back, and your shoulders. You may even continue on and fill your throat and your head before exhaling slowing and gently out through your nose as well.

3. If for some reason your nose is clogged, you may inhale and exhale through your mouth. However, breathing through your nose for this practice is infinitely more effective in leading you to the peace, stillness, and space deep inside your body.

4. When you notice your mind wandering while you are doing this practice, please simply say "thinking" to yourself, and then bring your attention and your awareness back to your body and your breath. When you find yourself thinking about anyone or anything, or talking to yourself in any way, very gently just bring your focus back to inhaling slowly, deeply, and fully.

5. Please do not judge, fight, or resist any of your thoughts or emotions. Simply and kindly say "thinking" when you notice you are not aware of your body or your breath and then shift your attention back to inhaling slowly, deeply, and fully.

6. In any moment, you can consciously choose to come back to your body and your breath, and in so doing, you will always find deep peace, space, and stillness underneath all of your thoughts and emotions.

7. Give yourself permission to let go and relax. Allow your body, heart, and mind to open and release any stress or tension you're holding. Allow your breath to melt and heal any blocks or pain that you feel in your body.

8. Repeat this practice as often as you can throughout the day. It can be done sitting, standing, or lying down for as long as you'd like. This practice is also great in the morning to wake you up as well as in the evening to relax your body, heart, and mind.

9. *Additional Step*: If you would like to take this meditation practice deeper, the following points will offer you structure and guidance to do so. Before you begin, I highly recommend finding a quiet place to sit where you will not be disturbed.

• *Creating Time and Space for a Consistent Meditation Practice:* Each time you practice your meditation, please decide on a specific amount of time you feel comfortable committing to your practice. I recommend beginning with ten minutes at first and then increasing your practice by ten-minute intervals each week until you can sit in meditation comfortably for at least one hour. Please also find an alarm on your clock, watch, or phone that you can use and set so you're not constantly checking the time. Once you do set the alarm and begin your practice, try not to check the time until the alarm goes off. Constantly checking the clock is just another subtle way of distracting ourselves from the present moment. Also, please put your phone(s) on silent so you won't be disturbed. Lastly, I highly recommend creating a consistent meditation practice in the morning before you leave your house, because it is the best way to create your day from a place of peace, positivity, and clarity.

- **Effective Meditation Posture:** Whether you practice on a chair, bench, couch, meditation cushion, or floor, please make sure you are sitting up straight and that your posture is tall and strong. You can sit back in your chair if this feels most natural; however, please make sure you're extending up through your spine so your vertebrae are not under too much pressure. At the same time, please relax all the muscles in your lower, middle, and upper back so there's no additional tension being created in your body. It's also helpful to imagine a string attached to the crown of your head that's gently pulling you up and taking the pressure off your spine. In regards to your head position, it's best to look straight ahead and then very slightly tilt your chin down.

   In regards to your legs and feet, if you are sitting on a chair, couch, or bench, it's best to have both feet flat on the floor, as this helps ground and balance the energy in your body. It's also helpful to have your knees at a ninety-degree angle so the energy and blood in your legs can flow freely. If your knees are too high above your pelvis, the energy and blood will get stuck around your hips and you'll feel uncomfortable while practicing your meditation. Thus, if you have long legs or are sitting on a small chair, this can be remedied by putting a pillow under you to boost you up a bit. If, on the other hand, your feet do not touch the floor for any reason, it's helpful to put a pillow under your feet. If you're sitting on the floor, or on a meditation cushion, it is best to have your legs crossed. Once again, it's ideal to have your knees lower than your pelvis so the energy and blood can flow freely without getting stuck. Thus, if your hip-flexors and groin muscles are tight, it's best to sit on a pillow or meditation cushion to ensure that your pelvis is higher than your knees.

In regards to the position of your hands, it is best to have them either palms down on your thighs or together in your lap in some way. If you have them together in your lap, I recommend gently interlacing your fingers. Ultimately, it's important to find a position that feels good for you so you can remain still throughout your meditation practice.

- *Eyes Open versus Eyes Closed:* The last key point to address in deepening your meditation practice relates to your eyes being either open or closed while you practice. Both approaches are very effective, and they both deserve equal attention. Practicing with our eyes open is very important because it helps us cultivate our ability to "be in the world" consciously without being reactive. Ultimately, we want to bring the peace found through meditation into our daily lives, so meditating with our eyes open helps us bring more presence, awareness, and love into every moment, experience, situation, and relationship. Practicing with our eyes closed is also important because it encourages us to go deeper into the peace, stillness, love, and awareness within us. It is very nourishing to close off completely to the outside world and then dive deeply into our body, heart, and soul.

When meditating with your eyes open, the best approach is to look down toward the ground about four to six feet, or one and a half meters, in front of you. When practicing with your eyes open it's best not to look at any one point in particular but rather to relax both your eyes and your gaze on the general area in front of you. When we fixate ("zoom in") on a particular point on the floor it's the same as fixating on a thought in our mind, so any time you find yourself fixating on a spot or piece of dirt on the floor, please treat this experience as a thought, say "thinking" to yourself, relax your gaze ("zoom out"), and then return your awareness to your breathing and your body. When meditating with our eyes open, it's best to direct 95 percent of our awareness inward and only 5 percent outward. The idea is to be visually aware of the 180-degree perspective in front of you while remaining fully aware of your body, breath, and thinking processes as well. In the beginning, this technique can feel a bit awkward, but in time it becomes more natural and leads to extremely deep levels of peace and self-awareness.

When meditating with your eyes closed, simply close your eyes and follow the next step outlined below.

- *Closing Points:* After finding the meditation posture that works best for you and setting your alarm, please follow steps one through seven from the simple deep-breathing meditation practice above **(page 89)**. After inhaling and exhaling slowly, deeply, and fully for a few minutes, please allow your breathing to become natural and uncontrolled. Then, please rest your awareness on your breath so you can observe each inhale and each exhale while simultaneously feeling your whole body. In deepening your meditation, please focus on steps four through seven from the practice above, but allow your breathing to be completely natural and unforced. As described in the steps above, when you find your mind wandering and notice yourself thinking about anything or anyone, please say "thinking" to yourself and then gently bring your attention and focus back to each inhale and each exhale and to feeling your whole body as you breathe.

In the end, there is no right or wrong way to practice your meditation. What matters is your commitment to (1) remaining present to all your thoughts, emotions, and physical sensations and (2) welcoming everything that arises with unconditional love, acceptance, and compassion.

While deepening your meditation practice, it's very helpful to know that physical irritation and discomfort often arise as blocks or sabotages to self-mastery and self-love. Most of us have a large amount of repressed psychological and emotional irritation and discomfort stored within us, which initially surfaces during meditation as physical agitation and restlessness before it can be healed. Thus, it is crucial to surrender and accept the physical discomfort that arises as you lengthen your practice because this is the only way to heal the underlying emotional discomfort that needs to be liberated before you can find lasting inner peace, health, happiness, and fulfillment. With this in mind, it is important to stay committed, persistent, and patient with your meditation practice even if agitation, irritation, or discomfort arise.

Lastly, I highly recommend rereading this particular chapter after you've practiced the above meditation a few times. It will continually offer guidance and clarity as you master loving yourself unconditionally and come home fully to life in the present moment.

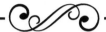

You are told to love your neighbor as yourself. How do you love yourself? When I look into my own mind, I find that I do not love myself by thinking myself a dear old chap or having affectionate feelings. I do not think that I love myself because I am particularly good, but just because I am myself and quite apart from my character. I might detest something which I have done. Nevertheless, I do not cease to love myself. In other words, that definite distinction that Christians make between hating sin and loving the sinner is one that you have been making in your own case since you were born. You dislike what you have done, but you don't cease to love yourself. You may even think that you ought to be hanged. You may even think that you ought to go to the police and own up and be hanged. Love is not [just] affectionate feeling, but a steady wish for the loved person's ultimate good as far as it can be obtained.

—C. S. Lewis

CHAPTER THIRTEEN

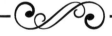

Love Yourself Unconditionally

What can we gain by sailing to the moon if we are not able to cross the abyss that separates us from ourselves?

—THOMAS MERTON

> *Wherever you are, please take a few slow, deep breaths into your belly. Please also feel your whole body, from your feet all the way up to the crown of your head, and then down to your fingertips. Please surrender fully and accept everything that you're thinking, feeling, and experiencing here in this moment. Please be present to your body and your breath.*

When we look closely at our relationship with ourselves we will see that most of us live in a way where we only love ourselves "if" and "when" we meet certain conditions that we've created for ourselves and then projected onto some distant future or some long-gone past.

- I will love myself "if" I'm in a loving relationship.
- I will love myself "when" I become successful.
- I will love myself "if" I lose weight.
- I will love myself "when" I make more money.
- I will love myself "if" I get that degree.

- I will love myself "when" I have that new car or that new house.
- I would love myself "if" I didn't have wrinkles.
- I would love myself "if" I didn't have this illness or this disability.

Does this conversation sound familiar?

Because most of us never learned how to love ourselves unconditionally, just the way we are, we constantly look to a fantasy reality in the future where we think we'll be more loveable, more deserving of love, or more able to love ourselves than we do right now. Less often, some of us even take this dynamic and turn it around by looking back on our past with regretful thoughts ("I used to love myself when ..." or "I would love myself if I looked like I did back when ..."). In these rarer cases our conditions are placed in the past, and this ultimately keeps us stuck in guilt, regret, or resentment over what has been and gone and therefore no longer is.

Regardless of where we place our conditions, if we continue to relate to ourselves in conditional ways, we'll never get to the future place or the past place where we're finally ready to love ourselves unconditionally here in the present. We have to begin to love ourselves here and now first in order to create, accomplish, and find what we desire most in life. It is never the other way around, despite how much we believe it to be so.

Looking to the future in order to love ourselves more in the present will never help us love what we have not been able to love already within ourselves, our lives, or our past. Similarly, holding onto situations, relationships, or images of the past that are loaded with regret or denial will never help us love and accept ourselves unconditionally or create healthy, happy lives here in the present either. What we do not love about ourselves, our lives, and our past in this moment will always remain beneath the surface of our awareness until we lovingly and honestly face it, accept it, forgive it, understand it, and therefore heal it. Regardless of how far or how much we try to run from or deny these challenging inner truths, they will constantly block us from the source of peace, health, happiness, fulfillment, and love within us, while they simultaneously drive us to create situations and relationships that are full of additional pain and confusion.

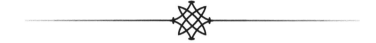

Our conditional love for ourselves is generally rooted in deep feelings, thoughts, and limiting beliefs around not being "enough" or "worthy of love" just as we are, which leaves many of us feeling we must always be more, do more, or have more to finally be loveable to ourselves and to others. At the core of this self-destructive internal dynamic is the fact that when we were growing up most of our parents could not love us unconditionally, just as we were, because they did not love themselves unconditionally just as they were. Thus, not only did we inherit a lack of self-love genetically at birth, but many of us were also raised in homes where no matter how much we tried to please our parents or make them happy, nothing would ever or could ever be "enough" to satisfy the insecurities, inadequacies, and expectations that they unconsciously projected onto us.

As a result, many of us have now lived a number of years believing that we're not good enough, smart enough, successful enough, attractive enough, and so on. We've also lived unaware that another way of life exists outside of our self-imposed limitations and conditions, one where we always feel connected to the inherent wholeness, abundance, and worth of our soul's true nature.

What most of us rarely hear, even now as "adults," is that not only are we all deserving and worthy of love—no matter what—but also, who we truly are beyond our limiting beliefs already is pure, purposeful love. That's why we all want and need love so deeply, and this is also why love, in its enlightened form, always feels so good and so liberating. We're all simply looking for the love that we are so we can just be the love that we are. In other words, we're all intuitively looking for ourselves so we can just be ourselves.

Because the larger majority of us remain unaware of this, however, we're still creating our lives from a mind-set of lack, unworthiness, and inadequacy. We constantly compromise and hurt ourselves for the love of other people, always trying to please them and keep them happy because we mistakenly believe this is still the only way to survive or get by. Meanwhile, our true needs, desires, and dreams continually get ignored because we don't think or feel that we're loveable, deserving, or worthy of having what we genuinely value or envisage for ourselves.

Fortunately, however, each of us is destined to wake up from this perceptual nightmare and then heal ourselves by letting go of the limiting conditions that we continuously place on our own love for ourselves here in the present moment. A key to achieving this is understanding that beneath all the limiting conditions we create or take on there is simply repressed emotional pain, which is the result of all the times in the past where we have not related to ourselves with the unconditional love, kindness, and compassion that we deserve.

Our limiting beliefs around being inadequate, unworthy, or undeserving in any way paradoxically exist to protect us from the uncomfortable emotions that we ourselves have created and stored within our body, heart, and mind. All the aspects of ourselves, our lives, and our past that are, or were, painful—that we judge, reject, deny, hide, run from, fear, feel insecure about, ashamed of, angry about, regretful for, or guilty about—are the only obstacles that block us from feeling and experiencing our soul's abundant true nature, which is always enough, always whole, and never lacking in anything.

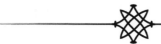

From a broader perspective, when our love for ourselves is conditional in nature, so too are the peace, happiness, and fulfillment that we experience on a daily basis. Underneath the conditions that we all place on ourselves as to "if" and "when" we'll finally be at peace, happy, or satisfied in life are really the conditions that we place on ourselves as to "if" and "when" we'll finally be loveable to ourselves and to others.

When we live believing that we'll only be loveable "if" and "when" we meet certain conditions that are not present here and now, we're in effect giving our peace, happiness, and fulfillment away to these external conditions, which always translates into not being at peace, happy, or satisfied now. In the same way that we search for love outside of ourselves when we do not love ourselves unconditionally, we also look for peace, happiness, and fulfillment outside of ourselves when we're not at peace, happy, or satisfied with *who we are, who we've been, or with the life we've created.* So, whether we're looking for love, or for peace, happiness, and fulfillment, we're always led back to mastering life's most important lesson—that is, loving ourselves unconditionally here in the present moment regardless of where we are, what we've done, or where we want to go.

It doesn't matter how many goals we achieve, how much money we make, how great our body looks, or how many good deeds we do; we will always find ourselves faced with the same parts of ourselves, our lives, and our past that we still do not feel good about or at peace with. Thus, our soul is constantly calling out for us to drop our limiting beliefs and conditions so we can face and feel everything within us that we fear and then honor, value, and love ourselves enough not to settle for anything less than the liberated, passionate, and joyful life that we know is our destiny and our birthright.

When we finally stop running from what we fear within ourselves, our lives, and our past, it's easy to see that we only create self-destructive conditions to protect ourselves and distract ourselves from what remains unhealed, unloved, and unexpressed within us. Furthermore, once we truly slow down enough to drop out of our head into the depth and wholeness of our being, we'll always find an ocean of love, peace, happiness, and fulfillment beneath all the negative beliefs and feelings that we hold within and toward ourselves. In this revelation comes a deep surrender, along with a clarity that sees every limiting condition that we place on our peace, happiness, fulfillment, and love for ourselves as just a pattern of thought that does not serve us anymore; one that is blocking us from the freedom and joy that are always available in this moment, regardless of what is occurring in the present or has occurred in the past.

Heal Yourself Now Questions

What conditions do you place on yourself as to "if" and "when" you will finally love yourself here in the present moment?

What conditions do you place on yourself as to "if" and "when" you will finally be at peace, happy, and fulfilled?

What stories do you tell yourself about why you are not loveable? What negative beliefs do you hold about yourself right now that block you from loving yourself unconditionally? What about you, your life, or your past justifies you feeling unworthy or underserving of love?

Do you always feel that you must be more, do more, and have more to finally feel loveable to yourself and to others? Do you always feel that you must be more, do more, and have more to finally be at peace, happy, or satisfied within yourself and your life?

Do you think your mother and father loved themselves unconditionally? If not, can you see that it was hard for them to love you unconditionally and to teach you how to love yourself unconditionally?

Do you feel you always had to be more, do more, or have more so your parents would love you or so they would be happy and satisfied with you? Can you see how your conditional love for yourself began at a very early age?

What can you focus your energy on today that represents you loving and valuing yourself and therefore honoring what you love to do, want to do, or need to do?

Love Yourself Now Affirmations

I am loveable just as I am. I am enough.

I do not need to be more, do more, or have more
to feel good about myself and my life.

I deserve love in my life. I always have and I always will.

I forgive my parents for not teaching me to love myself
unconditionally. I forgive my parents for not being able
to love, accept, and support me unconditionally.

I now choose to relate to myself with unconditional love, kindness,
and compassion in every moment, situation, and relationship.

The past and future are not real. All I ever have is now,
and all the love I need is already alive within me.

CHAPTER FOURTEEN

Welcome and Accept All of Who You Are

Out beyond our ideas of wrong-doing and right-doing,
There is a field. I will meet you there.
When the soul lies down in that grass,
The world is too full to talk about,
Language, ideas, even the phrase "each other" doesn't make any sense.

—JALAL UDDIN RUMI

Wherever you are, please take a few slow, deep breaths into your belly. Please also feel your whole body, from your feet all the way up to the crown of your head, and then down to your fingertips. Please surrender fully and accept everything that you're thinking, feeling, and experiencing here in this moment. Please be present to your body and your breath.

We all judge ourselves, and at times we all judge others. In both cases, our judgments exist merely to protect us from feeling the painful and uncomfortable emotions that we've repressed throughout our lives. Through judging other people we unconsciously, but only temporarily, make ourselves feel better about what we judge in ourselves. In other words, we only judge others to protect us and distract us from what we struggle to welcome and accept within ourselves and our own lives.

Ultimately, who we truly are beyond our own self-judgments is always whole and always loveable, regardless of what we perceive. Thus, when we judge ourselves to be inadequate, unlovable, or underserving in any way, the reality is we've merely lost touch with the truth of who we are, because beyond our limited perceptions of ourselves, our true self is far more abundant and loveable than we can even begin to imagine.

We all briefly forget the limitlessness of our soul's true nature, but eventually we're all destined to experience, feel, and know this deep inner truth once again. To find the psychological, emotional, physical, financial, and spiritual freedom that we're seeking, each of us is called to create a welcoming environment within ourselves so we can acknowledge and accept the many different aspects of ourselves, our lives, and our past. To liberate ourselves from our suffering and fulfill our life's purpose, each of us is challenged to open deeply to our most vulnerable inner truths, to both our "darkness" and our "light," and to surrender fully into embracing everything that we find.

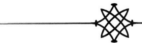

If we look honestly at the ways in which we relate to ourselves today, the majority of us will discover that there are many things within us that we judge, reject, deny, hide, and run from daily. In other words, most of us do not lovingly welcome and accept all of who we are or all of what we think, feel, want, and need. As we've seen before, these patterns around judging, rejecting, and denying our inner truths began building when we were very young, mainly because we feared losing the love and support we needed in our early years. To varying degrees, we all still carry these aggressive, fear-based patterns with us today. In fact, many of us have lived our entire lives totally unaware of how far we've moved away from who we really are because we never learned how to consciously welcome and accept all of ourselves all the time.

Once again, the root causes of the self-destructive relationship that we each have with ourselves to some degree go back to the very beginning of our lives, because this was when we learned to love and accept ourselves conditionally. You could say that even upon our conception and throughout our mother's pregnancy, we learned about the nature of love through the lens of unhealthy, limiting conditions.

Most of us were conceived in the energy of what our parents believed and felt to be love, both for themselves and for others, at that particular point in their personal growth and evolution. More specifically, when it comes to the relationship that our parents had with themselves at the time of our conception, it was most likely not the healthiest one, because this is true for most people. We could go so far as to say that the nature of the relationship we each have toward ourselves today was in the works long before we were even close to being conceived, with roots stretching way back biologically through our genetic line and spiritually through lifetimes worth of karma.

Ultimately, in this lifetime, the people who birthed us and raised us could not give us what they themselves were never given or had not learned for themselves. Our parents and most of the people who influenced us growing up did not accept themselves entirely, so logically it follows that they could not completely accept us or show us how to relate to ourselves in this kind and compassionate way—even if they truly wanted to or tried to.

Although this dynamic has been many people's experience, we still cannot afford to waste our time or our energy blaming our parents, or anyone else, for the lack of love we have for ourselves in the present. Our parents, along with every other person alive, struggled to welcome and accept themselves unconditionally, whether they were conscious of this inner reality or not. As human beings, we're all challenged by the inner relationship we have with ourselves, regardless of whether or not we express this vulnerable inner truth. Hence, we're all called to find a place of compassionate understanding within ourselves where we (1) release all blame and (2) accept all of who we are now.

And those who were seen dancing were thought to be
insane by those who could not hear the music.

—FRIEDRICH NIETZSCHE

We have all developed unconscious fears around being judged, rejected, and denied by other people because we fear feeling the emotional pain that we associate with these experiences. On a deeper level, however, we actually fear the emotional pain that we've created for ourselves by judging and rejecting ourselves so often in the past.

Instead of always being true to ourselves, most of us just continuously judge, reject, and hurt ourselves in the exact ways that we subconsciously fear being hurt by other people. We obviously don't realize it but this unconscious, self-destructive, and aggressive internal dynamic has created countless inner battles between who we really are and the person we've become in order to be loved, accepted, approved of, and supported throughout our lives. Thus, far more than losing love from other people, we really fear feeling all the repressed emotional pain that has built up within us over the many years of trying to be someone or something that we're not just to please other people.

Ultimately, the longer we go without fully accepting the wholeness of who we are, the longer we remain disconnected from our authentic true self and the more miserable and frustrating our lives become. To finally find the inner peace, health, happiness, and fulfillment that we're all seeking, we must learn to forgive ourselves for not accepting ourselves in the past and then be open to welcoming everything within us all of the time.

As young children, we didn't know how to accept ourselves or stick up for ourselves. But you and I are not small kids anymore, and we now have both the power and the awareness to face and feel everything that we've disconnected from within ourselves, our lives, and our past. We all have the strength as well as the courage that's necessary to consciously welcome, accept, and honor the wholeness of who we are.

Understanding the reasons why we never developed unconditional acceptance for ourselves to begin with is critical in learning how to accept ourselves unconditionally here and now. Being aware of how and why we disconnected from the love that we are, from our soul's true nature, ultimately helps us to remember and embody all of who we are once again. In understanding why we've never fully welcomed or embraced ourselves in the past, we finally empower ourselves to see the unhealthy, destructive, and aggressive ways we've been relating to ourselves for what they are so we can truly let them go.

Moving forward in our evolution as human beings is a process by which what is unconscious within us becomes conscious so we may grow and move beyond mere survival to thrive in harmony with all aspects of life. Another way of saying this is that our personal evolution, health, happiness, and fulfillment depend upon our willingness to welcome all that we have judged, rejected, denied, and hidden in the past.

Thus, in each moment that we choose to consciously accept and express all of who we are without allowing our fears or self-judgments to hold us back, we take a huge step forward in our personal healing and awakening toward living our most liberated and joyful life. If we can continually surrender into the truth of what we think, feel, want, and need in every moment, situation, and relationship without rejecting, denying, avoiding, or running from anything that arises within us or in our lives, we can easily accept, love, and reunite all the fragmented aspects of ourselves and our soul, and in so doing find the inner freedom, peace, and fulfillment that we deserve.

Heal Yourself Now Questions

What do you judge, reject, deny, or hide
about yourself in the present?

What do you judge, reject, deny, or hide
about your life in the present?

What do you judge, reject, deny, or hide about yourself from the past?

What do you judge, reject, deny, or hide
about your life from the past?

When you observe yourself with other people, what
do you typically judge about them? Can you see how
this mirrors what you judge about yourself?

What are your core insecurities right now? What
do you feel insecure about from your past?

What do you fear people knowing about you, your life, or your
past? Do you have any secrets that you hide from everyone or
from certain people? If so, who do you hide from and why?

If you could travel back in time and speak to yourself
as a child, what would you say to him or her in regards
to being true to yourself all of the time?

What can you focus your energy on today that represents
you loving and valuing yourself and therefore honoring
what you love to do, want to do, or need to do?

Love Yourself Now Affirmations

It's okay that I judge myself sometimes.

When I judge myself or other people, I'm
just protecting myself from pain.

I accept my whole self. I welcome my darkness and my light.

I do not need to deny my wholeness to be loved.

I am loveable just the way I am. I deserve
to be loved for who I really am.

I can live my life for me. I'm not here to please
others or to make them happy.

I am here to be myself and to enjoy my life.

I am one with God. I am one with the earth, with
all life, and with the entire infinite universe.

CHAPTER FIFTEEN

Forgive Yourself and Your Past Now

You who want peace can find it only by complete forgiveness.

—*A Course in Miracles*

> *Wherever you are, please take a few slow, deep breaths into your belly. Please also feel your whole body, from your feet all the way up to the crown of your head, and then down to your fingertips. Please surrender fully and accept everything that you're thinking, feeling, and experiencing here in this moment. Please be present to your body and your breath.*

Deep down we're all good, loving people, and yet we all live with things that we've said or done that we still struggle to forgive. Regardless of how bad, guilty, ashamed, angry, or regretful we feel about past situations, relationships, or decisions, we must eventually understand that each experience was ultimately awakening us to our true self and to the purpose of our lives.

If we have unconsciously acted in ways that have caused ourselves or others pain, it's always because we had lessons to learn so we could evolve and grow in a loving presence and awareness. Thus, the shame, guilt, anger, and regret that we still feel and store subconsciously within our cells hold jewels of wisdom that are waiting to teach us about what's most important in life—about truth, honesty, forgiveness, acceptance, and unconditional love.

If we do not open to accepting and eventually forgiving the things in our past that we still feel shame, guilt, anger, or regret around, then these aspects of our lives will always remain as inner blocks to us finding lasting inner peace, health, happiness, and fulfillment. On top of this, the toxic emotions that are tied up with what remains unforgiven will drive us to create additional experiences in which we feel negatively about ourselves and our lives. We'll just continually create painful experiences in the present until we realize that we're destined to forgive ourselves and move forward with our lives.

No matter how guilty, ashamed, angry, or regretful we feel, we're all both capable and deserving of forgiveness. Each of us deserves to be forgiven for the pain we've caused other people, but we will not be able to openly accept or receive this forgiveness until we're truly able to forgive ourselves. Even in situations where the person we've hurt has not forgiven us, we can still forgive ourselves, face the guilt or shame, grow from the experience, and then move on.

Everything that we experience in this life is meant for us to learn from, including what we perceive to be our mistakes. In fact, our so-called mistakes are actually the most important life lessons that we've needed to learn in order to grow and evolve toward our destiny and greatest potential. Loving ourselves unconditionally, therefore, requires that we come to understand the lessons inherent within the painful situations we've created, because this enlightened awareness is what allows us to untie the energetic knots of shame, guilt, anger, and regret that are connected to these past experiences. As we come to understand why we've acted or reacted in certain ways that have caused other people pain, we're then able to forgive ourselves and move forward with fulfilling our life's purpose to bring unconditional love into the world.

There's no doubt that at times it can be difficult to forgive ourselves when we've unintentionally hurt people we love or have loved deeply. But at some point, regardless of how much suffering we've caused, we have to come to forgive ourselves, because our repressed guilt, shame, anger, and regret will not only hold us back and keep us miserable, it will also create toxicity within every cell of our body and every relationship and situation in our lives. Thus, to free ourselves from our suffering we have no choice but to make peace with the pain we've created, because the only path to peace, health, happiness, and expanded awareness is one that's paved with humility and forgiveness.

Through forgiving ourselves we can finally heal what we've judged, rejected, denied, hidden, or avoided and thus reunite our inner world, which naturally frees us from our suffering and opens the space for love and compassion to shine through our every thought, action, and spoken word. Through forgiving ourselves we also grow in self-awareness, presence, and wisdom, which organically stops us from acting or reacting in unconscious ways that result in pain or suffering for ourselves or for others.

A person will be called to account on Judgment Day for every permissible thing he might have enjoyed but did not.

—THE TALMUD

Beyond forgiving ourselves for the pain that we've caused other people, we must learn to forgive ourselves for the pain that is at the source of all the pain we've ever created in our lives. Thus, with conscious awareness and unconditional love we must go back through each stage of our lives and forgive ourselves for compromising, abandoning, betraying, and hurting ourselves for the conditional love, acceptance, approval, and support of other people. Ultimately, we must go back in time and forgive ourselves for forgetting who and what we truly are, because this pain that we've been inflicting upon ourselves since we were children is actually the underlying reason for all the pain we've ever created for other people.

To find lasting inner peace, health, happiness, and fulfillment we all must eventually forgive ourselves for forgetting our soul's deepest inner truths. In other words, here in the present moment, we're called to open our hearts and to forgive ourselves for being so hard, so critical, and so aggressive with ourselves to the point that we could not welcome and accept the wholeness of who we are. Life asks each of us to exercise the inner compassion necessary to forgive ourselves for judging, rejecting, denying, and running from our inner truths so consistently throughout our lives.

Furthermore, we're also called to forgive ourselves for taking on external conditions as to "if" and "when" we'll finally love ourselves in our entirety. Our souls are crying out for us to forgive ourselves for all the pain, confusion, and frustration we've created for ourselves by relating to ourselves and to life from a place of fear. Finally, we're all challenged to love, accept, value, honor, respect, express, trust in, stick up for, and believe in ourselves so we do not hurt ourselves or others but rather create a healthy, happy, and fulfilling life where there's nothing to forgive ourselves for anymore.

Heal Yourself Now Questions

What in your life right now do you feel guilt, shame, anger, or regret about? Are you ready to forgive yourself now and move forward?

What do you still feel guilt, shame, anger, or regret about from your past? Are you ready to forgive yourself now and move forward?

Where do you still compromise yourself and abandon your inner truth? Are you ready to forgive yourself now and move forward?

Where have you compromised and betrayed yourself in the past? Are you ready to forgive yourself now and move forward?

Where do you still judge yourself in your life? Are you ready to forgive yourself now and move forward?

How are you still hard on yourself in your life right now? Are you ready to forgive yourself now and move forward?

Can you see how the only reason you've ever hurt another person is because you were hurting within yourself and thus avoiding the truth in some way?

What can you focus your energy on today that represents you loving and valuing yourself and therefore honoring what you love to do, want to do, or need to do?

Love Yourself Now Affirmations

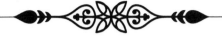

Deep down I know I am a good person.

Everything happens for a reason.

I forgive myself for the hurt I've caused myself and others.

I forgive myself for hurting (name the person(s) you've hurt).

My mistakes in life have been purposeful and necessary.

I forgive myself for not knowing how to love myself unconditionally.

My soul is pure unconditional love. I am here to forgive.

CHAPTER SIXTEEN

Forgive Others and Move On With Your Life

You will not be punished for your anger, you will be punished by your anger. Holding on to anger is like grasping a hot coal with the intent of throwing it at someone else; you are the one who gets burned.

—BUDDHA

Wherever you are, please take a few slow, deep breaths into your belly. Please also feel your whole body, from your feet all the way up to the crown of your head, and then down to your fingertips. Please surrender fully and accept everything that you're thinking, feeling, and experiencing here in this moment. Please be present to your body and your breath.

Ultimately, it is through learning to forgive ourselves that we grow in our capacity to forgive others. If, however, we have not welcomed what we see to be our own mistakes in life and therefore learned the purposeful lessons inherent within these experiences, then we will continuously struggle to forgive others for what we still perceive to be their own missteps, especially the ones we feel have hurt us personally. It's not until we truly forgive ourselves that we open to understanding that everyone is still learning and growing, including ourselves. Thus, as we deepen our own awareness into how and why we ourselves have created situations or relationships in the past where we've either caused ourselves or others pain, we simultaneously grow in compassion for other people.

Eventually we realize that the only reason why we ourselves or anyone else would ever create pain for another person is because deep down we're hurting inside and reacting to this hurt. Thus, as we come to understand our own choices and our own actions more deeply, we also gain insight into why others have acted or continue to act in ways that have caused, or still cause, us pain. And it is this new level of understanding other people that makes it possible for us to wholeheartedly forgive them.

Ultimately, in time, we all come to realize that we're no different and no better than anyone else, and to judge anyone as "wrong" or "bad," for any reason, is simply unconscious destructive behavior. Everyone, including you and me, is just looking for love, security, understanding, and happiness, even when we create chaos or pain in the process.

From a strictly self-interested perspective, forgiving others is actually much healthier than holding on to anger, resentment, or hatred, because these negative and aggressive emotions only eat away at our own health, happiness, and well-being. They also block us from moving forward in our own lives toward inner wealth, success, fulfillment, and freedom. This is why it's so important to face the anger, resentment, and hatred that we hold personally toward other people or groups, because whenever we allow ourselves to live with this pain for extended periods of time we're literally giving our life and our joy away through this subtle form of victimhood.

By offering justifications for why we shouldn't take complete responsibility for our own inner peace and happiness right now, we ultimately just make ourselves sick and miserable, regardless of how the person we expect to feel bad actually feels. However, when we finally find the strength, wisdom, and humility to forgive others and move on with our lives, we can easily reclaim our life and our power to create what we truly want and need most to fulfill ourselves and our life's purpose.

When another person makes you suffer, it is because he suffers deeply within himself, and his suffering is spilling over. He does not need punishment; he needs help.

—THICH NAHT HANH

Eventually you'll realize for yourself that in order to wholeheartedly love yourself, or, in other words, be free from suffering completely, you must embody the unconditional love that you are by bringing true forgiveness into this world. When it comes to forgiving other people, we're always brought full circle back to forgiving ourselves. Whenever we've experienced hurt in relation to another person or situation, it's almost always because we've allowed it to happen; it's nearly always because we were unaware to some degree, most likely compromising, abandoning, or betraying ourselves in some way for the love, acceptance, attention, or support of other people.

As difficult as it can be to swallow at times, we are never actually victims. If we still feel hurt by others for any reason, the heart of the issue always comes back to us not loving ourselves in some way. With this in mind, please love yourself, forgive yourself, and set yourself free. You didn't know any better. You were learning, just as we all are. Please also forgive everyone who you feel has hurt you in some way. They didn't know any better either. They too are still learning. Please allow these people to be free as well; in so doing, you'll not only be moving forward in fulfilling your own life's purpose, but you'll also find the peace, health, and happiness *that you deserve now.*

Heal Yourself Now Questions

Are there people in your life who you feel have hurt you, betrayed you, violated you, or wronged you in some way? Who are these people that you feel anger, resentment, or hatred toward, and why do you feel the way you do?

Have you forgiven these people completely for the pain you feel they have caused you? If not, why not? Are you ready to forgive them, forgive yourself, and move forward with your life?

Has anyone broken your heart whom you have not forgiven?

Do you hate anyone or anything? If so, who, what, and why? Can you see how underneath your hatred of others, there are things that you hate and have not forgiven in yourself?

Do you truly want to give your health, happiness, and peace away to the people who have hurt you in the past?

Can you see how in each situation and relationship where you've felt hurt or taken advantage of, you've actually compromised, abandoned, or betrayed yourself in some way? Can you forgive yourself for not knowing how to love, honor, and respect yourself?

What can you focus your energy on today that represents you loving and valuing yourself and therefore honoring what you love to do, want to do, or need to do?

Love Yourself Now Affirmations

Please make a list of every person whom you feel anger, resentment, hurt, or hatred toward. Then, please use their names with the following affirmation:

"I forgive (person's name), and I set myself free."

I forgive myself for being unaware. I forgive myself for not loving myself.

I am love, and love naturally forgives.

I too have acted in ways that have hurt other people. How can I not try to forgive?

I can forgive without being naïve. I can forgive and still honor myself and my inner truth.

I'm ready to forgive and move forward with my life's purpose.

I forgive myself for seeking other peoples' love, acceptance, approval, and support to my own detriment.

CHAPTER SEVENTEEN

Follow Your Big, Beautiful Heart

*If everyone approves of what you are doing, I urge
you to reconsider what you are doing.*

—Saint Germain

> *Wherever you are, please take a few slow, deep breaths into
> your belly. Please also feel your whole body, from your feet all
> the way up to the crown of your head, and then down to your
> fingertips. Please surrender fully and accept everything that
> you're thinking, feeling, and experiencing here in this moment.
> Please be present to your body and your breath.*

E very desire within our heart is the evolutionary impulse of life
and nature driving us forward toward our destiny and greatest
potential. The desires within our hearts are in fact the desires of God,
the desires of the intelligent universe, to know itself and express itself
more fully through our lives. There is no desire alive within us that
cannot become our reality, because *anything we truly want is predestined
to be realized in our lives.* In other words, there is nothing we desire
that we are not both capable and deserving of creating, having, or
achieving. We merely have to love and value ourselves enough not to
settle for anything less. Ultimately, every desire that we experience

contains a vital lesson we must learn in order to master loving ourselves unconditionally and thereby bring the unconditional love that we are fully into this world. All of our desires are in fact steps up the ladder, leading us toward our soul's ultimate desire for spiritual liberation and enlightenment.

Contrary to what is often taught, desire does not always lead to suffering. Desire only leads to suffering when we're attached to getting what we want because we're trying to avoid the truth in the present moment. Thus, when we can accept everything that is true both within us and around us, and also face our emotional wounds with courage, we can simultaneously feel the desire to create, experience, and achieve certain things without it leading to more suffering.

Desire that is free from denial and fear actually leads to joy and fulfillment. The evolutionary force of the universe, which is alive inside every one of our cells, is always guiding us forward toward the peace, health, and happiness we seek *through our desires*. Thus, regardless of how hard we try, the universe's desire to express itself through our physical existence cannot be stopped, ultimately because you and I are both one with, and also the result of, this creative force and intelligence that deeply desires to know itself and enjoy itself through everyone and everything that comes into being.

Even if what we desire initially causes us pain, ironically, it is the desire itself that eventually forces us to face the underlying causes of our suffering. If, for a period, we desire large amounts of pleasure merely to avoid what's difficult in our lives, at some stage we'll realize that our focus is not bringing the lasting inner peace, happiness, or fulfillment we thought it would. As we face this fact fully we can accept the uncomfortable emotions that we've been avoiding or numbing ourselves to, and then finally heal them and let them go.

This process naturally gives rise to a purer form of desire, which then guides our every movement forward toward fulfilling our life's purpose. If, however, we continually deny what we desire, regardless of our reasoning, we just end up repressing the life and the love that are trying to live and express through us. By rejecting our desires, we unintentionally reject the lessons and the healing that our desires are driving us toward. Thus, it is always in our best interest to go after what we truly want and to learn the liberating lessons that our soul is craving to learn.

Whether our initial desire is for food, alcohol, drugs, sex, money, attention, fame, recognition, love, or freedom, going after it, even if it causes us pain, is better than constantly denying the desire's existence, because it's only through excessive craving for anything or anyone that we eventually find balance and learn to value moderation and self-discipline. Like a bird that continually flies into a glass window and hurts itself because it does not see the window, we too must go after things that create pain before we naturally choose not to and feel at peace with our choice.

To truly free ourselves from suffering, we also have to go after what we desire so we can see through the illusion that it will somehow make us happy or fulfill us. There's no way around this unless we trap ourselves in a cave, and even then most of us won't truly find what we're looking for. Through following our heart, we eventually realize exactly what we need to realize about what supports our overall well-being and love for ourselves, and what does not, because it's only through trial and error that we finally learn to enjoy life each day without doing so self-destructively. This dance between what we desire and the associated pleasure and pain always leads to a clear understanding of the universe's perfectly designed plan to (1) wake us up and (2) help us remember that all of the peace, health, happiness, fulfillment, freedom, and love we desire will only be found in the depths of our own heart and soul.

Finally, we cannot repress our desires in hopes of avoiding pain, because we can never free ourselves from suffering by avoiding our suffering. Our liberation is only found by courageously stepping into the heart of our pain with unconditional love for ourselves. Thus, we are called to (1) feel into the core of our suffering so we can uproot it completely and (2) always follow our inner voice, because as we do so, the love within us naturally heals and fulfills our deepest wounds from the inside out.

Even when masked by self-destructive and pleasure-seeking behavior, our desires will eventually bring us to our knees in surrender, to a higher truth, because our heart is forever guiding us to love ourselves, others, and all life unconditionally even if we hurt ourselves to some degree in the process. In the end, every desire will indeed lead us to wisdom, enlightenment, and freedom.

Love has no other desire but to fulfill itself.

—KAHLIL GIBRAN

Each of us ultimately wants to thrive in life as a free and full expression of who and what we truly are. I'm sure you would agree that your heart's deepest desires are always to feel good, to feel love, to feel joy, to feel free, to feel whole, to feel abundant, to feel at peace, to feel safe, to feel fulfilled, to feel inspired, to feel vital, to feel connected, to feel understood, and to feel valued, respected, and appreciated for who you truly are.

In any moment that *we do not feel these qualities* in our life experience, it is a clear indication that we need to honor ourselves, follow our heart, and love ourselves more deeply in some aspect of our lives. Any time that we feel negative, anxious, unhappy, unsatisfied, insecure, fearful, lacking, incomplete, empty, angry, resentful, frustrated, rejected, guilty, ashamed, regretful, lonely, or unwell, in any way, our soul is crying out for us to follow our heart, heal our pain, and go after what we truly want and love in life.

Even when we doubt ourselves, our heart will always persist in directing us forward toward a life that fully reflects the joy, wisdom, and love that are inherent to who we really are. Thus, regardless of how strongly we try to deny it, our soul's inner voice will never stop pointing us toward (1) where we're meant to be and (2) what we're meant to be doing.

The primary reason why so many of us do not follow our heart all of the time is once again because of who and what we fear. Like we've seen before, we all fear feeling the emotional pain that must be transformed in order to break free from our ego's protective shell. We also fear the unknown territories that our heart and soul are guiding us into, because moving forward requires us to change and grow beyond our current state of being and way of life. Ironically, many of us even fear experiencing life in positive ways because we've never known any better or any different. Many of us actually fear being healthy, happy, and satisfied on a regular basis, because consistently living in such a high vibration and state of consciousness is such a foreign experience. As much as we're curious, most of us are still afraid of what exists outside our current comfort zone.

Sometimes we fear feeling guilt about letting go of a job or a relationship that does not reflect what we truly want for ourselves or our lives any longer. Other times we fear the grief and the pain of experiencing loss or of feeling alone in the world. Quite often, we fear hurting other people when we make a decision to honor ourselves and follow our heart's inner guidance because sometimes the direction of our growth takes us away from people who are, or have been, very important to us. Beneath our fear in these situations, however, lives that same fear of feeling the emotional pain that we ourselves have created in all the past moments where we have compromised and abandoned ourselves by not following our heart's inner guidance.

Rather than face these emotions as they arise within us, many of us just stay in the situations and relationships that we're not satisfied or happy with because we're not prepared to take responsibility for what we're really feeling. It is so important to understand that when we fear hurting another, we're most often just afraid of facing what will arise within us once we actually let go of whatever doesn't reflect our true needs or desires at a particular point in our lives. Our fears arise within us, and then our mind kicks in to justify and rationalize why we should stay where we're miserable ultimately just to avoid facing the implications of making the choices that are now necessary to move forward on our destined path.

Whatever course you decide upon, there is always someone to tell you that you are wrong. There are always difficulties arising which tempt you to believe that your critics are right. To map out a course of action and follow it to an end requires courage.

—RALPH WALDO EMERSON

One of the biggest excuses that so many of us use not to honor the guidance of our hearts is that we're scared of how others will judge us and of what others will think of us. When we react in this way we allow our fears to control our lives and we end up hurting ourselves because we're not prepared to take full responsibility for our own health and happiness.

What we often fail to realize is that trying to please everyone around us is the quickest path to depression, resentment, and dis-ease. By continuing to (1) judge ourselves or (2) fear the judgment of others, we end up denying and rejecting our heart's inner guidance, and we once again create tremendous suffering on top of the pain we're already trying to free ourselves from. Ultimately, what other people think of us and how others judge us is not our problem. As long as we're coming from love and taking personal responsibility as we honor ourselves, without unconsciously causing other people pain, what we do with our lives is up to us and no one else.

It's very liberating to know that the only reason why another person would ever judge us in the first place is because they judge themselves. And the only reason why they judge themselves is because they do not feel good about something in their own lives. Through judging us they unconsciously protect themselves from whatever remains unhealed and unloved within them. So, whenever you feel judged, or fear being judged, all you have to do is be true to yourself, accept yourself, and keep in mind that other people's judgments are not actually personal in any way.

Ultimately, as we master loving ourselves unconditionally we also master following our inner guidance without worrying about or fearing what other people will think. When we truly respect the heartfelt force deep within us, we not only love ourselves more for it, but we also realize that denying its guidance just creates suffering and unhappiness. We eventually realize that our own self-judgments and fears are the only obstacles really holding us back and everything else is just another excuse to complain or play the victim. In fact, when we stop judging ourselves and finally break through our fears, we don't attract judgment from others nearly as much, and when we do, we're simply too busy enjoying our lives and fulfilling our life's purpose to notice it.

All our dreams can come true if we have the courage to pursue them.

—WALT DISNEY

Tied up with our fear of being judged is also our fear of failure. Many of us deny our heart's inner voice so often because we're afraid of making the "wrong" decision or of changing our mind somewhere along the way. *What will they think of me? What if I do not or cannot follow through? What if I decide I want or like something different? What if I'm not good enough, smart enough, or strong enough?*

Even if we fear failing at something, we will always feel better for trying, regardless of the outcome. The true failure is in not trying at all, in not going after what we want and love with all of our heart and soul. In the end, success is not defined by achieving a goal; it's defined by the courage and strength that we find within ourselves, which then leads to inner peace, fulfillment, and self-respect.

Through following our heart each day we naturally build belief and faith in ourselves, because the more consistently we honor our inner guidance, the more we trust it is leading us where we're meant to go. This process organically deepens our confidence in ourselves, which just snowballs with every step we take toward fulfilling our desires, passions, and dreams.

Thankfully, we cannot make a wrong decision, because every time we follow our heart we experience exactly what we're destined to experience for our soul's growth, evolution, and liberation. If we find ourselves desiring something different at any point, there's absolutely nothing wrong with choosing a new direction, because as we become more aware we also become more clear about what we want, need, and value. It is always better to take the risk, to jump, to try, to learn, and to grow than it is to become paralyzed by who and what we fear. It is always better to live, explore, and love than to suffer silently with regret.

Life is not really about where we end up; it is about how fully and authentically we live each moment and each day. Thus, if we achieve a goal but have betrayed our inner truth anywhere along the way, we will never *feel the success* we're looking for. We can only succeed in life when we follow our heart and therefore know, in every cell of our body, that we've been true both to ourselves and to others. When our lives are built upon the inner success that is born from loving ourselves and living with integrity, we not only free ourselves from our suffering, we also discover that the foundations of our daily existence have become so strong that we'll never fear failing in anything our heart inspires us toward ever again.

Heal Yourself Now Questions

In your heart, what do you want and need right now?

What do you want to feel, experience, create, do, and accomplish?

Whom or what are you allowing to stop you?

Who or what are you afraid of? Whose judgment do you fear?

Whose approval do you self-destructively seek?

What stories are you telling yourself that are really
just excuses to mask your fear of failure, fear of
judgment, or fear of feeling emotional pain?

Are you ready to move beyond your stories and
your fears? If not today, then when will you?

Do you want to live a life that is defined by regret?

Love Yourself Now Affirmations

I deserve to be happy.

When I follow my heart, everything always works out for the best.

The desires in my heart are God and the
universe guiding me forward.

I create all that I desire with ease.

My heart is one with God's heart.

My heart is one with every human heart.

Love is my ultimate desire.

As I follow my heart, I heal my heart and find the love I'm seeking.

What other people think of me is not my concern.

I have all that I need within me to create a fulfilling life that I love.

CHAPTER EIGHTEEN

Choose Love over Fear Always

The cave you fear to enter holds the treasure you seek.

—JOSEPH CAMPBELL

> *Wherever you are, please take a few slow, deep breaths into your belly. Please also feel your whole body, from your feet all the way up to the crown of your head, and then down to your fingertips. Please surrender fully and accept everything that you're thinking, feeling, and experiencing here in this moment. Please be present to your body and your breath.*

Intentionally channeling the love that we are toward healing the fear within us is a key to loving ourselves unconditionally. Our psychological, emotional, physical, financial, and spiritual freedom depend upon our willingness to (1) live in the present moment and (2) choose to focus our beliefs, thoughts, emotions, actions, and spoken words on love. Consciously focusing on love, on giving love to ourselves, on giving love to others, on thinking about love, on thinking about whom we love, what we love, what we love to do, as well as on what we *would love to do, feel, and experience* is what guides us toward the joy and freedom we're seeking in every aspect of our lives.

In every moment of every day we make choices, either consciously or unconsciously, that shape the quality of our lives, our relationships, and our overall wellbeing. When we make a conscious choice we make a choice based on love: love for ourselves, love for others, and love for our planet. When we make an unconscious choice we make a reactive choice based on fear: fear of survival, fear of pain, fear of losing control, fear of losing love, or fear of losing our sense of self, or who we think we are.

Liberating ourselves from our suffering demands that we choose consciously as much as we can in every moment, situation, and relationship, and choosing consciously always entails choosing love in the face of fear. To choose love, we're constantly called back to life here in the present moment so we become more aware of the inner processes by which we're shaping and creating our lives. Most importantly, our soul's innate intelligence is guiding us home to our deepest inner truths so we can recognize the fear-based tendencies that are stopping us from creating the healthy, happy, and fulfilling lives we all deserve.

As we deepen our awareness in every moment, situation, and relationship, we begin to see clearly that beneath every unconscious or self-destructive choice we make there lives a fear-based reactive pattern that's occurring within our body, heart, and mind. As we awaken to these internal defense mechanisms, we also begin to realize that if we do not transform these fearful reactions within us, we will constantly project them out onto our perceived future and thereby create a life that is not only defined by what we fear, but also one that completely reflects our fears as well.

Fear that is not honestly faced and transformed in the present moment will always drive us to create the exact situations and experiences that we fear most, thereby reaffirming our fear-based limiting beliefs while simultaneously sabotaging our health, our happiness, and everything else potentially positive in our lives. By living in the present moment, however, we can bring the light of our conscious awareness deeply into our fears and thus illuminate what is actually true both within us and around us in the here and now. As we do this we naturally come to understand that (1) our current fears have their roots in the past and (2) we do not have to project these past fears onto our future—especially when we're fully conscious of them.

As we become more aware of the fear-based, limiting beliefs that we hold, we can see how our experiences of the past shape and limit what we believe our experiences of the future can and will be. Hence by bringing more awareness to this very moment, we can liberate ourselves from the painful and confusing experiences we create because of fear and thus stop limiting the amazing opportunities each new day presents. Ultimately, the more grounded we are here in the present moment, the less we project our fears of experiencing what we have in the past onto the future, and the more space and energy we leave available for us to create our lives from a place of love and unlimited possibility.

Our deepest fear is not that we are inadequate. Our deepest fear is that we are powerful beyond measure. It is our light, not our darkness that most frightens us. We ask ourselves, who am I to be brilliant, gorgeous, talented and fabulous? Actually, who are you not to be? You are a child of God. Your playing small doesn't serve the world. There is nothing enlightened about shrinking so that other people won't feel insecure around you. We were born to make manifest the glory of God that is within us. It is not just in some of us: it's in everyone. And when we let our own light shine, we unconsciously give other people permission to do the same. As we are liberated from our own fear, our presence automatically liberates others.

—Marianne Williamson

Practically speaking, there are two main ways to transform the fear inside of you and liberate yourself from this unconscious emotion that (1) protects you and (2) holds you back in life. Both of these approaches depend first upon you living in the present moment.

1. ***The first way to transform your fear is to get it out by writing about it or by talking about it with a trusted person in your life.*** We do not often share our deepest fears with anyone, not even ourselves, because we either deny that they exist or we judge ourselves for feeling fear in the first

place. When we judge ourselves for having fears, most of us then project our own judgment of ourselves out onto others, which just leads us to fear being judged by other people. Thus, whether we deny our fears or judge ourselves for having them, they then remain trapped within us, subconsciously driving our choices in every moment and creating additional separation and limitation in our lives.

However, as we begin to write about our fears or express them to someone we feel safe talking to, we begin to see through our fears and thus liberate the life force energy that has become trapped in the ongoing loop of fear within us. Honestly facing and expressing our fears immediately breaks this cycle and allows us to reclaim our vital life force energy from the destructive patterns of denying our fears or judging ourselves for having them.

Ultimately, when we live with deeply repressed fears and do not express them in some way, we unconsciously allow them to rule our lives, because anything inside of ourselves that we resist will always persist and grow in the shadows of our body and our subconscious mind. Through denying, rejecting, and avoiding our fears, they do not go away; they just expand in power and destructive influence. In other words, anything that we do not honestly, lovingly, and consciously face within ourselves or our lives will haunt us until we do. Thus, when we fight our fears, we unintentionally feed them and make them grow.

2. *The second way to transform your fear is to focus on love— to consciously and intentionally choose love as much as possible each and every day.* As I mentioned above, focusing our beliefs, thoughts, emotions, actions, and spoken words on love is integral to loving ourselves unconditionally, to liberating ourselves from suffering, to fulfilling our life's purpose, and to realizing our full potential. When we train our mind to focus on whom we love, what we love, what we love to do, and also on what we would love to do, have,

and experience, we are focusing our vital life force energy on creating what we want and need most to construct a fulfilling life that we love.

What we focus on grows in the same way that what we resist persists. So focusing on what we love feeds energy into the manifestation of more things to love in and about life. Many of us are unaware of this and therefore do not choose to focus on what we love enough. Rather, we focus a lot of time and mental energy on the things in and about our lives that we do not love, and in so doing we unintentionally cause these things to grow in our experience.

Even though experiencing more of what we do not want in life is the last thing anyone would consciously choose, many of us are trapped in this self-destructive and self-defeating pattern of relating to ourselves because we don't know anything different. Rather than consciously expressing our fears and choosing to focus on all that we love each day, we unintentionally allow our fears to simmer and stagnate, which just causes us to feel negative about ourselves and our lives—essentially because we're unconsciously giving our vital life force energy, joy, and power over to (1) whom and what we fear and (2) what we do not want to experience.

By living as presently as possible, however, we can all learn to love ourselves and reclaim our power, joy, and life force energy from the fear we allow to hold us back. Once we find the courage to face our fears fully, our vital life force energy is finally free and available to channel toward consciously creating the life we truly desire. Thus, once we're actually aware of the destructive, limiting influence that fear has on our lives, we can choose to express our fears without letting them fester, because we know it will set us free. We can also choose to focus on whom and what we love as much as possible, because when it comes down to it, what else really matters?

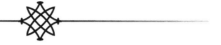

The contrast in our experience between feeling love and feeling fear is always guiding us forward toward our destined liberation. Ultimately, without experiencing fear, we could not know just how liberating the experience of loving ourselves, loving others, and loving life truly is. Our fears are actually gifts that challenge us to love ourselves unconditionally in every moment, situation, and relationship so we may free ourselves from our suffering and fulfill the purpose of our lives.

Ironically, our greatest fears always become the bridge to our most liberated and joyful life. They always end up strengthening our commitment to our destiny because they consistently teach us to choose love over fear, no matter what, which is the only way to create a beautiful life that is full of honesty, peace, health, happiness, fulfillment, and deep heart-to-heart connection. Thus, every time we love ourselves enough to make a conscious choice grounded in love, we awaken more fully to the facts that (1) we are pure love, (2) our soul is eternal, (3) God lives in us, as us, and (4) we already have everything we need to free ourselves from all forms of suffering. As we remember these deeply empowering inner truths, we simultaneously realize that we do not need to fear rejection, death, punishment, or pain, because we're already united with the source of all love, our soul will never die, we cannot make a mistake, and deep down, we've always known that our suffering is merely leading us home.

CHAPTER NINETEEN

Rediscover Your Faith and Trust

As soon as you trust yourself, you will know how to live.

—JOHANN WOLFGANG VON GOETHE

> *Wherever you are, please take a few slow, deep breaths into your belly. Please also feel your whole body, from your feet all the way up to the crown of your head, and then down to your fingertips. Please surrender fully and accept everything that you're thinking, feeling, and experiencing here in this moment. Please be present to your body and your breath.*

Our faith and trust in ourselves, in our life's purpose, in life itself, in the universe, and in God are challenged and tested each and every day. We are constantly called to honor the voice of our heart and soul and to break through our fears, our doubts, and our self-imposed limitations. Our rational mind may say, "But how can that work out?" or "That's what I want and need, but I don't think it's possible," or "I don't deserve that." But even in these moments, deep in our heart we still know that it is possible to do, have, create, and experience what we desire most in life. Deep down, our soul knows that the love inside of us is strong enough to break through every internal and external barrier to make possible what we feel to be our destiny and our birthright.

Our lives would be significantly easier if we had learned that there is a fundamental perfection to life that permeates all of nature and the entire universe. In other words, we would all be able to accept ourselves, our lives, and our pasts unconditionally and thus be completely at peace, if we truly knew that everything is always as it is meant to be, even if we do not fully understand it or like it.

If we cannot see and feel this perfection unfolding within our lives right now, it's only because we have not healed and therefore understood the emotional pain that still lives beneath our fear-based resistance and lack of acceptance. This emotional pain is really the only obstacle that blocks the unshakeable faith and trust that's already alive within each of us. Most of us have merely forgotten the fact that we ourselves have created our lives in order to bring the love that we are fully into this world. We've also forgotten that one hundred percent of our unhappiness, anxiety, and sickness stem from all of the times in the past where we have not related to ourselves with the love, kindness, and respect that we deserve.

Any struggle that is present in our lives right now is in fact the exact obstacle we need to face and transform in order to heal and move forward in fulfilling our life's purpose. In other words, the lessons around loving ourselves unconditionally that we are here to master are present within the aspects of ourselves and our lives that we're currently not at peace, happy, or satisfied with. Once we accept that everything is always exactly as it is meant to be, we can allow ourselves to trust that we're exactly where we need to be, doing exactly what we need to be doing, in order to master the lessons necessary to create a fulfilling, healthy, and prosperous life.

Most of us were never taught that our lives are embraced by a larger, universal story that is (1) much bigger than our individual lives and (2) always unfolding both within us and all around us. However, once we expand our perception on life to include the universe's ever-present perfection, we can finally open to trusting life wholeheartedly *just as it is* without constantly projecting fear, anxiety, negativity, and regret onto each moment and situation.

It is so liberating to know that everything that occurs in our lives occurs exactly when it's supposed to, without any exceptions. Everything that has ever occurred and everything that will ever occur is a part of a larger natural order that we must learn to accept and cooperate with if we genuinely want to find lasting inner peace, health, happiness, and fulfillment.

In the same way the seed of a rose bush sprouts roots, grows upward from the ground, and eventually flowers in its own perfect time, our own destiny, healing, and liberation unfold exactly as and when we're ready. A butterfly cannot break free from its cocoon until it's strong enough to see the whole process through in the same way a human baby generally takes nine months to gestate before its body, organs, and entire being is ready for its new life in the outer world. In other words, we can never force an organic process and truly achieve a positive, harmonious outcome. All life naturally contains an inner awareness, or intelligence, that knows exactly when it's time to take the next evolutionary step.

> *I have been away from my own soul too long, so late sleeping,*
> *But that dove's crying woke me and made me cry.*
> *Praise to all early waking grievers!*
> *Some go first, and others come long afterward.*
> *God blesses all in time… how to say this to one who denies it?*
> *We are all made of the sky's cloth, and everything is soul and flowering.*
> *Everything is soul and flowering.*
> *Everything is soul and flowering!*

—Jalal Uddin Rumi

The primary reason why so many of us do not have faith and trust in ourselves, in our life's purpose, in life itself, in the universe, and in God right now is because we know that in the past we have not related to ourselves from a place of unconditional love, kindness, and compassion. We know that in the past we have hurt ourselves by compromising ourselves, by abandoning ourselves, by not valuing ourselves, by judging ourselves, by disrespecting ourselves, by not believing in ourselves, by not sticking up for ourselves, and by not honoring and expressing our deepest inner truths. Quite simply, many of us do not have faith and trust in ourselves, because we keep betraying ourselves by giving away our personal power, happiness, and security to other people in exchange for their conditional love, acceptance, approval, and support.

Would you agree that if your own best friend or your intimate partner continuously betrayed you, you would most likely find it very difficult to trust them again?

Well, you and I were intended to be our own best friends, so when we betray and hurt ourselves in the ways that we do and have done, we make it quite difficult for us to trust ourselves. The only way to reignite our faith and trust in ourselves, in our life's purpose, in life itself, in the universe, and in God is to forgive ourselves and then commit to loving ourselves in every moment, situation, and relationship. Our soul is crying out for us to value ourselves enough to heal the pain we've created for ourselves in the past and to master rebuilding our lives from a place of fearless love for ourselves in the present. The evolutionary force of the universe is calling out for us to embody the love that we are so we can unlock the gates to our greatest psychological, emotional, physical, financial, and spiritual freedom.

Ultimately, we're all born with an inherent faith and trust that cannot be broken or taken away. It's like a seed of knowing and confidence within us that is just waiting to blossom and fill our being and our life. Once we stop compromising ourselves for other people's love, acceptance, approval, and support, our faith and trust in ourselves naturally strengthens, which leads us to remember that we've both chosen and created all of our life experiences to awaken the love, peace, and joy within us fully. As we stop giving our personal power away to other people and to external circumstances, we're then free to give ourselves the love we need for the faith and trust within us to expand infinitely. Eventually, through this process the seeds of unwavering clarity, certainty, and confidence within us burst wide open and fill every cell in our body and every experience in our life. Finally, through giving ourselves the love we need to blossom and thrive we remember that everything is, always has been, and always will be perfect just the way it is.

Including ourselves.

Heal Yourself Now Questions

Do you struggle to believe in yourself? If so, why?

Do you struggle to trust yourself? If so, why?

Do you struggle to trust others? If so, who?

Who in your life mirrors back to you your own self-doubt?

In other words, who doubts your abilities and capacities?

Where in your life are you betraying yourself and your truth?

Where in your life are you dishonest with yourself?

Where in your life right now are you being
dishonest with other people?

Which situations do you struggle to accept as purposeful
and necessary for your healing and growth? Can you see
how you have unintentionally created or allowed these
situations to develop? Can you forgive yourself?

What do you need help with in your life right now? When you
have some space, please write a letter to the universe or to God
asking for support with the situations and relationships in your
life that are challenging, confusing, overwhelming, or scary.

What can you focus your energy on today that represents
you loving and valuing yourself and therefore honoring
what you love to do, want to do, or need to do?

Love Yourself Now Affirmations

Being honest with myself is the key to my freedom.

Being honest with other people is the path to peace.

I forgive myself for betraying myself.

I forgive myself for betraying others.

I am committed to loving, honoring, and valuing myself.

I want to trust myself again.

I must trust myself to truly trust other people.

I must be honest with myself to be honest with others.

I must believe in myself before others will believe in me.

My outer world is always a reflection of my inner world.

I am always supported, protected, and safe.

Thank you God, and thank you universe, for your support.

Everything is exactly as it is meant to be.

CHAPTER TWENTY

Please Be Kind to Yourself

The softest things in the world overcome the hardest things in the world.

—LAO TZU

> *Wherever you are, please take a few slow, deep breaths into your belly. Please also feel your whole body, from your feet all the way up to the crown of your head, and then down to your fingertips. Please surrender fully and accept everything that you're thinking, feeling, and experiencing here in this moment. Please be present to your body and your breath.*

Are you your own worst enemy or your own best friend? Most of us are our own worst enemies. But to liberate ourselves from our suffering, we all must become our own best friends. In order to find the abundant source of peace, health, happiness, fulfillment, and love within the depths of our own being, we're all called to develop a deep respect for ourselves where we relate to ourselves with loving-kindness and compassion in every moment, situation, and relationship.

On our journey through life all of us become frustrated, angry, and severely dissatisfied at times. We all experience periods where we're truly unhappy with where we are in life and with what we've accomplished. If we're honest with ourselves, just about all of us will admit that sometimes we believe, think, or feel we should be further along than we are—happier, healthier, wealthier, more purpose driven, more successful, and so on.

I'm sure you can also relate to the fact that most of us are extremely hard on ourselves; we tend to be quite critical and aggressive with ourselves as opposed to being loving, kind, honest, and compassionate, like a true friend would be. Ultimately, when we find ourselves unhappy or unsatisfied with where we are in life, with what we're doing, or with our current situation it is a clear indication that we're not loving ourselves as deeply as we can in some aspect of our lives.

It is extremely common to feel displeased both with ourselves and with life at times. But it's precisely at these points that it is necessary to recognize the vital need we all have to relate to ourselves with more kindness and therefore accept the frustration, anger, and dissatisfaction we feel as essential and purposeful inner prompts that are guiding us to commit even more deeply to our purpose and path in life.

Like all things in life, how we feel during these periods of negativity and contraction will pass, and we will eventually open to the inner freedom, joy, and clarity we're seeking again, because these qualities are not only inherent to who we truly are, they are also always present within us beneath our suffering and unhappiness. In fact, the frustration, anger, and dissatisfaction that we experience are actually healthy and necessary reminders of the times in the past where we have not loved, valued, and honored ourselves, but rather compromised, abandoned, and hurt ourselves. These challenging emotions and the associated psychological tension are once again just cries from our soul asking us to bring more love and more kindness into our body, heart, and mind now.

Be soft. Do not let the world make you hard. Do not let pain make you hate. Do not let the bitterness steal your sweetness. Take pride that even though the rest of the world may disagree, you still believe it to be a beautiful place.

—KURT VONNEGUT

In bringing this gentleness to the very core of our being, we're naturally guided to move through the deepest and darkest places within ourselves. To reach the point where we truly love all of who we are, as well as all of who we have been in the past, we have to come face-to-face with our most challenging skeletons and demons. It is here where we befriend the deepest aspects of our unconscious self and heal the gap that's developed between who we really are and the false self we created to protect ourselves and survive.

Hence, bringing true compassion into our lives means we stop trying to be someone and something that we are not. It means we stop living our lives to please other people and we start honoring what we feel we need to fulfill our life's purpose and realize our greatest potential. Becoming our own best friend means we both value and accept our inner truths no matter what; it means we live from our heart, we follow our heart, and we always express ourselves honestly.

Through relating to ourselves with the deep kindness we deserve, we finally allow ourselves to relax into the present moment, into just being with ourselves, fully as ourselves, without having to be more, do more, have more, or be different from how we naturally are. We finally give ourselves permission to (1) stop beating ourselves up, (2) surrender into the unfolding of our destiny, and (3) just accept, appreciate, and enjoy where we are today.

Heal Yourself Now Questions

How are you hard on, critical of, or aggressive with yourself?

How are you hard on, critical of, or aggressive with other people? This will reflect how you relate to yourself.

What areas of your life are you frustrated with right now?

What are you angry at yourself about?

In what ways do you punish yourself?

Are you ready to forgive yourself and move forward?

What can you focus your energy on today that represents you loving and valuing yourself and therefore honoring what you love to do, want to do, or need to do?

Love Yourself Now Affirmations

If I am not for me, then who will be for me?

I am doing my best.

I don't exist to please others.

(Your name), I am here for you.

I will treat myself with the love, kindness, and respect that I deserve.

Additional Practice: Write a Letter to Yourself as Your Own Best Friend

When you have some space, I highly recommend writing a letter to yourself as if you were speaking to your own best friend. If your best friend was struggling with what you're currently struggling with in your life, what would you say? What encouragement would you offer? What wisdom or advice would you give?

CHAPTER TWENTY-ONE

Love Your Body, but Know You Are So Much More

To be beautiful means to be yourself.
You don't need to be accepted by others. You need to accept yourself.

—THICH NHAT HANH

> *Wherever you are, please take a few slow, deep breaths into your belly. Please also feel your whole body, from your feet all the way up to the crown of your head, and then down to your fingertips. Please surrender fully and accept everything that you're thinking, feeling, and experiencing here in this moment. Please be present to your body and your breath.*

L oving our physical body is undoubtedly a key to loving all of who we are, and because so many of us struggle to love our physical body, addressing this issue is a necessary step in transforming our suffering. Our physical appearance is often the one thing that determines what we think and how we feel about ourselves more than anything else in life, ultimately because we've all forgotten that while who we are includes our physical body, we are in fact far greater than what we see when we look in the mirror. Thankfully, once we begin to love ourselves unconditionally, we start to remember and identify with our ever-present inner beauty, which is never lacking or deficient in any way. But until we reach this felt awareness deep within ourselves, many of us are constantly fixated on trying to look different from the way we currently do, and this constant state of non-acceptance is at the heart of much of our suffering.

Anything about our physical body that we do not love right now is merely a reflection of something within us, our life, or our past that we have not learned to love unconditionally. In other words, any perceived physical imperfection or insecurity is merely a symptom, or a cry from our soul, asking us to love and heal some aspect of our nonphysical being more fully.

Most of us mistakenly identify with the reflection of ourselves that we see when we look in a mirror, but when we truly stop to consider and feel whether or not we are merely our physical body, the logical conclusion, to some degree, will always end up being; obviously not. The truth is that our physical body is an energetic expression of our soul in the same way that our thoughts and emotions are also energetic expressions of our larger and deeper self. In the same way branches, leaves, and fruit are natural expressions that grow from the trunk, or core, of a fruit-bearing tree, so too are our thoughts, emotions, and physical body just natural expressions of a much grander consciousness, soul, and spirit at the heart of who we are.

Who we truly are is actually an infinite source of energy, beauty, and love that is united with the entire intelligent universe. Our soul is united with every other soul as well as the one great soul of God. Even if we're not aware of this, the truth remains that our soul is what fills, shapes, and drives both the structure of our physical body as well as its life-giving functions. Our soul's true nature is also inherently loving, perfect, and beautiful, even when the beliefs we hold, the thoughts we think, and the feelings we feel in relation to our physical body say otherwise.

It is no measure of health to be well adjusted to a profoundly sick society.

—JIDDU KRISHNAMURTI

Ultimately, the relationship that we each have with our physical body was "shaped" by the unique familial, educational, cultural, and media influences that we encountered throughout our lives. But underneath all of the negative beliefs we might hold in relation to our physical appearance, or body image, we will always find emotional pain from past experiences, situations, and relationships that we have not fully felt or healed.

As we've seen in previous chapters, all of the pain, insecurity, unhappiness, and dissatisfaction we experience and hold will always lead us back to the moments and situations where we have not related to ourselves with unconditional love, kindness, and compassion, either because we didn't know how to or because we were afraid to. This internal dynamic always leads us to judge ourselves and judge our physical body, to some degree, in order to protect ourselves from feeling the unhealed emotions that are still stored within us. Thus, regardless of why, how, or what we judge about our physical body, it's always an issue of misperception, meaning that we're either completely identified with our physical body or, we're just attached to limiting beliefs about our physical body that definitely do not reflect our true nature, but which are very effective in protecting our hearts.

Whether we judge ourselves as being overweight or underweight, too small or too big in some part of our body, unattractive, imperfect, or disabled in any way, the truth is we've become attached to limiting beliefs and perceptions simply to protect us from feeling the uncomfortable emotions stored within us. The same is also true for every form of addiction that influences how we look and feel physically. Whether we're addicted to food, alcohol, cigarettes, drugs, sex, money, attention, misery, or being sick, underneath all our self-destructive habits, there's simply emotional pain that we're reacting to, numbing ourselves to, and subconsciously protecting ourselves from feeling.

As in all cases, the key to loving our physical body is to come home to the present moment so we can face and feel the underlying emotions that are (1) causing us to judge our physical body, (2) causing us to abuse our physical body, and (3) creating the physical symptoms and imbalances that we're experiencing. Thankfully, as we heal the repressed emotions that currently block us from loving our physical body, the love and beauty that are inherent to every soul naturally arise within us and guide us to care for our body and speak to our body with unconditional love all of the time.

The first step in changing anything is always complete acceptance of what is present. Therefore, once we finally accept what we do not love about ourselves both physically and non-physically, we actually empower ourselves to move in the direction that we truly want to go. When we do not accept our physical body just as it is, however, we just create more pain and misery for ourselves, because whenever we fight what is, we unconsciously choose to stay stuck in it. Thus, when we're finally ready to surrender our inner fight and wholeheartedly accept ourselves completely, we open the door to heal both our physical self-judgments and the underlying emotional pain, which then clears the way to intentionally create and achieve whatever we want or need to personally look and feel great.

Nothing ever goes away until it teaches us what we need to know.

—PEMA CHODRON

Ultimately every physical judgment, criticism, and insecurity comes back to our need and desire for love. Having grown up around people who did not love and accept themselves unconditionally, most of us did not receive all of the love and acceptance we needed as children. On top of this, we all inherited multiple forms of self-sabotage genetically from our parents, because they could not help but pass on their unhealed dysfunctions. For example, if one of our parents struggled to feel beautiful, then we were most likely born with the same limiting perception of ourselves already activated within our consciousness. Likewise, if we had parents who were very hard on themselves, then they were most likely just as hard on us. This makes it easy to see how over time most of us just end up internalizing our parents' criticism and judgment and literally walk around with their voices in our head.

Hence, underneath every physical self-judgment, self-criticism, and insecurity we will always find emotional pain that was first inherited and then built upon very early in our lives. *This is why so many of us feel as though we* were *just born feeling insecure, overweight, or unattractive.*

This underlying negativity is always the result of (1) <u>emotions and beliefs that we absorbed in our mother's womb between our conception and our birth</u>, (2) us not knowing how to love ourselves as children, (3) our parents not loving themselves unconditionally, (4) our parents not being able to love us unconditionally, (5) our current patterns around repressing what we feel, and (6) from a spiritual perspective, our soul's karma and core lessons in this lifetime.

Fortunately, no one has to live feeling negative about him or herself physically forever because through loving ourselves now we can transform all of the inner obstacles to feeling good about ourselves. No amount of physical judgment, insecurity, or negativity is too much to transmute into a healthy and positive inner relationship with our physical body. Not only does our true nature always remain beautiful, loveable, and whole beneath our limiting beliefs and perceptions, but also, we are all capable of loving ourselves in a way where we can heal and achieve anything we truly desire.

The degree to which we experience the positive feelings we crave depends upon how honestly we're willing to face ourselves and our lives. If we're prepared to love, honor, and value ourselves in the present, and also channel this love toward healing our past emotional hurt, there is nothing that is outside our power to transform. With patience and commitment, each of us can take full responsibility for relating to ourselves with love, for caring for our body each day, and for living a healthy, balanced, and proactive lifestyle while we heal our old emotional wounds and intentionally recreate our lives.

When it comes to loving our physical body completely, many of us are just waiting to be loved unconditionally by someone else. We're unconsciously looking to be loved, accepted, and supported in the ways we were not loved, accepted, or supported as children. Knowing this, it will never matter how much another person loves or accepts us if we do not embrace ourselves fully from the inside out. Each of us must eventually realize that we are the person we're waiting for, we are the love we're looking for, and we already have all the love we could ever ask for within our own heart. Ultimately, it is up to us to cultivate the inner discipline that's necessary to relate to our whole being with loving-kindness, because it's only through making this commitment each day that we allow the seeds of self-love, self-confidence, and self-respect to crack open and grow strong and permanent within us.

Heal Yourself Now Questions

What do you struggle to love or like about your physical body?

What are you insecure about physically?

Can you feel that you are so much more than just your physical body? Can you feel the life force energy vibrating within you?

If you look into your eyes in the mirror can you see that you are much greater than just your physical body?

What are you waiting for (if *waiting* metaphorically equals "carrying extra physical weight") to go after what you want and love? What are you waiting for to finally commit to achieving your goals? Whose love, understanding, approval, acceptance, or support are you waiting for? What if you never get it?

If you overeat, can you see how you're just numbing yourself to uncomfortable emotions?

If you feel excessively overweight, can you see how subconsciously you've built a physical shell to protect your heart from being hurt?

If you struggle with anorexia can you see how you are over identified with your body and looking for love externally?

Are you ready to be happy and love yourself from the inside out?

If you struggle with bulimia can you see how you are (1) looking for love, joy, and pleasure and (2) trying to numb yourself to your emotions?

Are you ready to be happy and love yourself from the inside out?

What did you need to hear as a child about your physical appearance but never heard? If you could tell your younger self anything right now, what would you want him or her to know?

If you think about past experiences where you felt insecure, unloved, or unattractive, what did your younger self need to hear or know to feel good about himself or herself in that moment or situation?

If you could go back in time and stick up for yourself as a child, what would you say and to whom would you say it?

Are you ready to commit to caring for your body? Are you ready to make lifestyle choices that are free of guilt? Are you ready to eat healthy, exercise regularly, and heal your destructive thoughts and negative self-talk?

Love Yourself Now Affirmations

It's okay for me to feel beautiful.

(Your name), you are beautiful just as you are.

I love and appreciate my body for supporting me and my life.

I am not just my body. I am so much more.

Thank you, body. Thank you, bones. Thank
you, organs. Thank you, cells.

Thank you for my healthy, flexible, beautiful body.

Thank you for my strong immune system. Thank you for my
strong digestive system. Thank you for my strong circulatory
system. Thank you for my strong reproductive system.

I accept my body as it is, and I commit to
caring for my body's health daily.

My body is a temple for my soul. It is my temporary home.

I am one with the soul of all life. I am one with the soul of God.

I am one with the infinite universe.

My body is a cell in God's body. I am a cell in the universe's body.

I am an infinite source of healing energy and love.

I am eternal and immortal. I was never born and I will never die.

Additional Self-Love Body Practice

Speaking to your body with love, kindness, and positivity on a regular basis will help you replace your negative thoughts and self-judgments. Thus, many of my clients (both male and female) have found it helpful to use the above affirmations while moisturizing their entire body either after showering or after bathing. Even if it's challenging at first, and even if you do not believe what you're saying completely, please be patient with yourself and persist, because in time you will allow yourself to open and receive your own loving support.

CHAPTER TWENTY-TWO

Practical Nutrition and Lifestyle Guidance Based on Self-Love

Be careful about reading health books. You may die of a misprint.

—MARK TWAIN

> *Wherever you are, please take a few slow, deep breaths into your belly. Please also feel your whole body, from your feet all the way up to the crown of your head, and then down to your fingertips. Please surrender fully and accept everything that you're thinking, feeling, and experiencing here in this moment. Please be present to your body and your breath.*

Considering that there are thousands of books about nutrition, exercise, and caring for your body, it's unnecessary for me to go too deeply into the physical aspects of loving your body. I'm sure you're well aware of what this entails. For our purposes, I will briefly share what I've found to be the most important and most effective approaches to loving your body from the perspective of creating a healthy and balanced lifestyle that is based on unconditional self-love.

Please keep in mind that all of us are slightly different when it comes to what's best for our body type, inner nature, and even the unique climate we live in. Overall, however, there are some key guidelines I've found to be generally supportive and loving for every-body. Having said that, I personally recommend and live by the following physical approaches to unconditional self-love.

- Try to drink a good amount of clean water (at least two to three liters) each day to flush out toxins in your body and to stay hydrated. Try to drink only natural spring or mineral water. There are also numerous filters available that you can buy for your home to filter the water from your taps.

- Try to drink at least two cups of water in the morning before you eat or drink anything else. This hydrates your cells, wakes up your organs, flushes out toxins, activates your digestive system, and helps your whole body function optimally throughout the day.

- Try to eat unprocessed, organic whole foods as much as possible. Whole foods such as vegetables, fruits, lean meats, wild fresh water or saltwater fish (as opposed to farm-raised), legumes, and whole grains. Once again, everybody is unique, so you have to find the combinations that work best for you.

- Try to avoid genetically modified foods.

- Also try to avoid foods containing preservatives, artificial colorings, and artificial sweeteners.

- Find a high-quality daily multivitamin from your local alternative health care practitioner. Other nutritional supplements that are generally great for all people to take daily, no matter what age or state of health, include high-grade fish oils, probiotics, and some form of green super food, such as spirulina or blue-green algae.

- Try to avoid eating large amounts of processed flour in breads, pastas, cereals, pastries, and cakes.

- Try to avoid eating fast food and processed meat.

- Try to avoid eating too much dairy in the forms of milk and cheese, because these foods create phlegm, stagnation, and blockages in our body and energy system. They also decrease mental clarity and sharpness.

- Try to avoid eating too much sugar in the forms of candy, soft drinks, and processed juices.

An American monkey, after getting drunk on brandy, would never touch it again, and thus is much wiser than most men.

—CHARLES DARWIN

- Try to avoid drinking too much alcohol.
- Try to avoid smoking.
- Try to avoid prescription and recreational drugs.
- Try to exercise in some way each day, even if that means taking a few short walks around your neighborhood or block. Walking, running, hiking, biking, yoga, qi gong, tai chi, weightlifting, dancing, and swimming are all great ways to move your body and your energy to keep yourself strong and well. Find something active that you enjoy and do it regularly.
- Considering the last point, although housework undoubtedly requires a lot of energy, it is not the same as taking time specifically to focus on loving yourself and caring for your physical health!
- Sexual intimacy is very important for most people. If you have not chosen a life of celibacy for religious or spiritual reasons, then regular sexual intimacy is healthy for your body, heart, and soul. Bringing a great deal of presence, awareness, communication, and respect to this part of our lives is also very important in our overall healing and spiritual awakening.
- Take time just to *be*, whether through meditation, reading, writing in a journal, taking a bath, listening to music, or making yourself a cup of tea. Allow yourself time and

space to simply be without having to do anything or be anywhere.

- Try to love yourself when you dress for your day. Whether you're going to work, out with friends, family, or your partner, how you dress does affect how you feel. Wear clothes that truly make you feel good about yourself and your life.
- Many deodorants and toothpastes contain chemicals called parabens, which are horrible for our health. Please find a natural deodorant and toothpaste to use daily.
- Also, a number of shampoos, conditioners, and other body care products are full of chemicals that are not good for our health. Some to avoid are sodium lauryl sulphate, sodium laureth sulphate, propylene glycol, and triethanolamine.
- Try to get between seven and nine hours of good sleep each night.
- With that in mind, if you're a coffee drinker, try not to have coffee within five hours of going to bed.

The greatest of follies is to sacrifice health for any other kind of happiness.

—ARTHUR SCHOPENHAUER

When considering the above-mentioned approaches to loving and caring for your body, please remember that moderation is always the best approach. Even moderation in being moderate is healthy once in a while too! The "middle way" tends to be optimal, as extremes of any kind throw us out of balance and often snap back with equal force the opposite way.

Please also remember that being kind toward yourself, regardless of your nutritional and lifestyle choices, is the top priority. If it takes you a while to truly love your body and relate to your body with love, then so be it. There's no need to suffer in the process. Life is too short.

CHAPTER TWENTY-THREE

Master Loving Yourself within Your Relationships

My primary relationship is with myself- all others are mirrors of it. As I learn to love myself, I automatically receive the love and appreciation that I desire from others. If I am committed to myself and to living my truth, I will attract others with equal commitment. My willingness to be intimate with my own deep feelings creates the space for intimacy with another. As I learn to love myself, I receive the love I desire from others.

—Shakti Gawain

> *Wherever you are, please take a few slow, deep breaths into your belly. Please also feel your whole body, from your feet all the way up to the crown of your head, and then down to your fingertips. Please surrender fully and accept everything that you're thinking, feeling, and experiencing here in this moment. Please be present to your body and your breath.*

Cultivating joyous, loving, and supportive relationships is one of the most important ingredients for living a healthy, happy, and fulfilling life. But today many of us place more value on things like achieving worldly success, always being right, making a lot of money, or projecting a certain image of ourselves out into the world. In focusing on these less valuable and superficial aspects of life over and above our precious personal relationships, we not only neglect our soul's most important and most liberating life lessons, we also pass up some of the deepest heartfelt and soul-nourishing experiences available to us as human beings.

All of our relationships are sacred blessings that offer us priceless opportunities for the healing, growth, and happiness that we're all looking for. Regardless of the external form a relationship takes, we always come together with other people to learn about love and compassion, to awaken and expand in awareness, to heal the wounds of our heart, and ultimately, to master loving ourselves unconditionally so we may bring the love that we are fully into this world.

Each and every relationship in our life right now is meant to help us transform our limiting beliefs so we may break through the inner obstacles that separate us from the kindness, peace, and joy that we're all meant to experience and share within our relationships to one another. The limiting beliefs that we hold about ourselves and our lives always conceal painful unhealed emotions, which, once healed, reveal that no one ever exists separately or apart from anyone or anything, regardless of how different or isolated we may feel.

Ultimately, we cannot and do not heal alone. Thus our personal relationships offer infinite potential and possibility for our healing and inner growth, because not only do they expose our unconscious limiting beliefs and unhealed emotional pain, but they also inspire and bring forth the love within us more powerfully than any other aspect of our lives.

Along with the flowering of this love, the aspects of ourselves, our lives, and our past that we still do not love unconditionally inevitably arise to be transformed within our relationships, because the love within us must eventually force out whatever remains unprocessed and unhealed inside us. Our current relationships, therefore, are the most influential catalysts on our healing and spiritual journey. The people in our lives are mirrors that reflect back the blind spots within our own self-awareness, ultimately helping us to love ourselves and grow in ways that are not possible outside of relationship. Thus, as challenging as some of our relationships might be, the people in our lives truly are our greatest teachers.

> *Self-love is the foundation of our loving practice. Without it our other efforts to love fail. Giving ourselves love we provide our inner being with the opportunity to have the unconditional love we may have always longed to receive from someone else.*

—Bell Hooks

Most of us do not see our relationships in such a positive light because our close relationships have often been, or still are, the most difficult and most painful aspects of our lives. Our close relationships are frequently painful experiences because they (1) reveal our pain-filled wounds from childhood, which resulted from us not receiving all of the love, attention, kindness, and emotional support we needed, and (2) they also mirror back the unhealthy, aggressive, and self-destructive relationship that many of us have maintained with ourselves throughout our lives.

With these points in mind, our current relationships to other people can only be as healthy as our relationship currently is with ourselves. In other words, the amount of love, respect, kindness, compassion, and happiness that we experience in our interactions with other people is a direct reflection of the amount of love, respect, kindness, compassion, and happiness that we currently feel within ourselves.

From this perspective, each person in our lives actually reflects back to us an aspect of ourselves that we're being called to love, value, and embrace. This is demonstrated by the fact that if we do not accept, appreciate, honor, trust in, or believe in ourselves, here in the present moment, then most of the people in our lives will not either. As we master loving ourselves within our current relationships, however, we not only find that the people in our lives reflect back to us the deep love, respect, and faith we've cultivated in ourselves, but we also find that who we are and what we embody inspires others to do the same for themselves.

If we truly want to be free from our suffering, we're eventually forced to recognize that when we relate to the people in our lives, we either relate to them consciously from a place of love and respect for ourselves or, we relate to them unconsciously from a place of fear, insecurity, and inadequacy. When we relate to others from a place of self-love and respect, we give and relate genuinely from a place of clarity, integrity, and peace, which means we do not have an inner conflict occurring as to whether we should or should not give of ourselves in some way. This means we give freely of ourselves without expecting anything in return, without placing conditions on what we give or do, and without manipulating based on what we've given or done either.

Loving ourselves unconditionally within our relationships also means we do not act or speak just to please others or to make them happy. It means we're always honest with ourselves and with whomever we're relating to, even if they want or expect something different or something more from us.

Conversely, when we relate to others from a place of fear, insecurity, or inadequacy, we tend to give and relate out of feelings of obligation or out of a fear of losing their love, a fear of hurting them, a fear of being hurt by them, or a fear of feeling guilty for saying no. When we come from fear, insecurity, or inadequacy, we act and speak merely to please others, and we end up compromising and abandoning what we truly think, feel, want, and need for ourselves in exchange for their conditional love, approval, acceptance, and support, which only leads to more pain, frustration, anger, and resentment.

Pause now to ask yourself if it is worth paying so much for so little. Imagine you say to the person whose special love you want, "Leave me free to be myself, to think my thoughts, to indulge my tastes, to follow my inclinations, to behave in ways I decide are to my liking." The moment you say those words you will understand that you are asking for the impossible. To ask to be special to someone means essentially to be bound to the task of making yourself pleasing to this person. And therefore to lose your freedom... Maybe now you are ready to say, "I'd rather have my freedom than your love." If you could either have company in prison or walk the earth in freedom all alone, which would you choose? Now say to this person, "I leave you free to be yourself, to think your thoughts, to indulge your tastes, to follow your inclinations, and to behave in any way you decide is to your liking." In saying those words to another, to any other, to your beloved —in saying those words you have set yourself free. You are now ready to love. For when you cling, what you offer another is not love but a chain by which both you and they are bound. Love can only exist in freedom. The true lover seeks only the good of the beloved which requires especially the liberation of the beloved from the lover.

—ANTHONY DE MELLO, *THE WAY TO LOVE*

In learning to love ourselves unconditionally it quickly becomes clear that much of our suffering is the result of us betraying ourselves in our relationships. All of us hurt ourselves within our personal interactions to some degree, because we falsely believe that if we please others and make others happy then they will please us and make us happy in return. Eventually, however, often after much pain and confusion, we realize that no one can ever truly bring us lasting happiness or fulfillment besides ourselves. We also realize that no matter how much we do for or try to please another person, at the end of the day, it will never be enough to fulfill them or make them happy.

From this perspective, it becomes pretty obvious that what most of us tend to call love is really just a subtle form of manipulation that is so common we've all convinced ourselves it's the "real thing." Betraying ourselves to meet the needs of another person, just so that person will love us in return, is not true love. Similarly, expecting someone to compromise him or herself just to satisfy all our personal preferences, merely as a prerequisite to us expressing love or affection toward them, is extremely misguided when it comes to the quality of love that we're all actually looking for.

As much as we sometimes think it to be so, the people in our lives do not exist merely to fulfill our own personal needs and desires. Nor do we exist merely to meet their needs and wishes either. For the most part, that was our mothers' and fathers' role during our early years, not our partners', our friends', or our children's responsibility now. Ultimately, each of us is destined to master fulfilling our own needs by giving ourselves the unconditional love, attention, and support that we (1) did not receive as children and (2) now unconsciously look for from other people.

At some point on our healing and spiritual journey, we're all forced to realize that achieving lasting happiness and fulfillment is always dependent upon the quality of love present within our own relationship with ourselves. Thus, if we truly want to create healthy, supportive, and conscious relationships that last, we must first create a healthy, supportive, and conscious relationship with ourselves. Likewise, if we genuinely want to experience true, unconditional love with another human being, we must first commit to finding the source of true, unconditional love within us, which is only possible through loving ourselves unconditionally in every moment, situation, and relationship.

Heal Yourself Now Questions

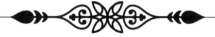

In which relationships do you struggle to love, accept, forgive, honor, value, respect, express, and stick up for yourself? Why do you feel you struggle with this?

Whom in your life do you find it hard to accept as your teacher?

Whom do you expect to make you happy, heal you, rescue you, take care of you, or fix you?

Whom do you try to make happy, please, fix, heal, or rescue?

With whom in your life are you codependent? In other words, whom do you betray yourself for and expect to do the same in return?

What can you focus your energy on today that represents you loving and valuing yourself and therefore honoring what you love to do, want to do, or need to do?

Love Yourself Now Affirmations

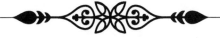

I am love, and I do not need to fear losing love.

I am enough. I am loveable just the way I am.

My health and happiness are in my own hands.

Every person in my life is my teacher.

It's never too late to start over.

It's never too late to love again. I'll never
be too old for love and romance.

I deserve intimacy and deep connection.

When I'm healthy and happy in myself, I naturally
create healthy and happy relationships.

My relationships are only as healthy as I am.

I deserve healthy, happy, and loving relationships in my life.

Additional Practice for Attracting a Life Partner or Soul Mate

1. Please make a list of all the qualities you would like in a life partner. Please list all of the character traits as well as all of the physical traits you desire. Then, please list everything you would like to do, create, feel, and experience with this person.

2. Once the above list is complete, please turn your request into a letter or prayer to the universe or to God and ask for what you want. "Dear God (or universe), please send me my soul mate who … Thank you for my soul mate who is …"

3. Once steps one and two are complete, please close your eyes and imagine what life will look like and feel like when you meet the person you're looking for. Please visualize what you will do, create, feel, and experience with this person. Then, in your heart, give thanks to the universe or to God for sending you your teacher, lover, and best friend.

4. Finally, after completing steps one through three, please focus on loving yourself, be patient, and be open to whomever you meet. It's very helpful to reread your letter or prayer often and to repeat step three as much as possible until he or she shows up in your life.

Additional Practice for Healing Your Current Relationship(s)

If you are struggling with any relationship in your life, whether it's with your partner, spouse, parent, child, or friend, it is very helpful to write the person a letter expressing how you feel, what you want, and what you need. At first, I recommend you write a draft of the letter that you will not give to them so you can express yourself fully without holding back. Then, it is helpful to rewrite the letter a second time with more clarity and personal responsibility, and with less reaction and blame.

In your letter(s), I recommend you use nonviolent phrases such as:

- I feel ... (hurt, angry, unappreciated, used, loved, respected, valued, etc.)
- I need ... (space to be, clear communication, respect, honesty, passion, etc.)
- I want ... (to do things I enjoy, have fun, share emotionally, travel, etc.)
- I feel hurt, angry, frustrated, or unvalued when ...
- I love it when you ...
- I appreciate it when you ...
- I need to feel safe, that I can trust you, that I matter, etc....
- I want to go, do, create, experience, etc....
- I want us to honor and respect what's important to each other...
- I'd like to be able to ...
- It's important to me that ...
- I really value or need some "me" time.

Underneath everything that we feel and desire there are important needs that must be met for us to (1) have a healthy relationship with ourselves, (2) have healthy relationships with others, and (3) be at peace, happy, and fulfilled. Thus, if we can learn to identify what we're feeling and desiring, and then recognize the underlying need, we can express ourselves from a place of clarity, love, and personal responsibility.

Another extremely helpful approach to healing a relationship with someone close to you is to ask them what they feel, want, and need. Oftentimes, we do not even know what we're feeling, desiring, or needing because we never learned how to be this present or clear with ourselves or with those around us. Thus, if you can help the people in your life to understand themselves more deeply in this way, there's nothing that cannot be overcome, healed, or harmonized for the benefit of everyone involved.

With the above in mind, when writing your letter(s), you can ask the person you're addressing what they feel, want, and need, in addition to expressing your own position. This particular approach opens a space that will help both you and the other person move forward with peace, understanding, and mutual respect.

CHAPTER TWENTY-FOUR

All Love Is Ultimately Self-Love

A human being is part of a whole, called by us the "universe"—a part limited in time and space. He experiences himself, his thoughts, and feelings, as something separated from the rest—a kind of optical delusion of his consciousness. This delusion is a kind of prison for us, restricting us to our personal desires and to affection for a few persons nearest us. Our task must be to free ourselves from this prison by widening our circles of compassion to embrace all living creatures and the whole of nature in its beauty.

—ALBERT EINSTEIN

Wherever you are, please take a few slow, deep breaths into your belly. Please also feel your whole body, from your feet all the way up to the crown of your head, and then down to your fingertips. Please surrender fully and accept everything that you're thinking, feeling, and experiencing here in this moment. Please be present to your body and your breath.

Ultimately, when we love and help ourselves we are also loving and helping other people, as well as all life on our planet, because in reality we are all one interdependent and interconnected web of life. The same is also true for when we give love either to other people or to other forms of life. Anytime we love or help another person or life form, we are in fact loving and helping ourselves, because there's no separation between us and anyone or anything that exists in the entire universe.

Once we truly love ourselves unconditionally, however, loving anyone or anything "outside" of ourselves actually becomes a *conscious process* of expanding our own love for ourselves. The important distinction to make here is that once we love ourselves unconditionally, *we actually become capable* of sharing love consciously, without conditions, as opposed to unconsciously "giving" love to others merely because we feel insecure, inadequate, or unlovable, or because we want, need, or expect something in return.

Even after all this time, the sun never says to the earth, "You owe me."
Look what happens with a love like that; it lights up the whole sky.

—HAFIZ

From the largest possible perspective, the entire universe can be viewed as one big body, or one self, and each of us can be seen as a cell in this universal body. From this perspective, all love is actually self-love, because everyone and everything is a part of this universal self. Another way of understanding this is that the universe is synonymous with God, and in the same way that we're all a part of the universal self, each of us is also a part of God's self. Thus, our own soul, what we perceive to be our individual "self," is both one with as well as a unique expression of God or the universal self.

From this viewpoint, the universe can also be seen as a system that functions solely on love for itself. If you think about the sun's light and energy that nourish life on our planet, we have a perfect example of universal self-love. All life on earth would cease to exist if the sun did not constantly and unconditionally express its love toward our planet. Trees, plants, fruits, vegetables, and grains would not grow from the earth. Humans and animals would have nothing to eat. The water we drink would remain frozen and undrinkable. All the trees and plant life would not receive the necessary sunlight and energy to convert carbon dioxide from the atmosphere into the oxygen we all need to breathe.

Life on this planet would clearly not exist if it were not for the sun's unconditional love for the aspect of itself that is the earth and all life upon it. Thus, as much as we perceive ourselves to be separate from the world around us, we can never truly separate ourselves from anyone or anything that exists, regardless of how hard we try.

If you love yourself, you love everybody else as you do yourself. As long as you love another person less than yourself, you will not succeed in loving yourself, but if you love all alike, including yourself, you will love them as one person and that person is both God and man. Thus he is the great righteous person who, loving himself, loves all others equally.

—MEISTER ECKHART

Another great example of self-love in the universe exists between a mother and her child. Most mothers actually love their children far more than they love themselves. In fact, many mothers give of themselves unconditionally to their children, even to their own detriment. Many mothers do this because they inherently know their children's lives are not separate from their own. Most mothers know in their hearts, whether they are conscious of it or not, that once they bring another life into the world, a large part of their purpose is to unconditionally love and nurture this life.

A parent's love for his or her child is one of the most powerful examples of unconditional self-love found in nature. In fact, the instinctual drive in both men and women to procreate is the evolutionary impulse of the universe awakening an unconditional love for itself through all forms of life.

One of the primary reasons why we actually have children is to master loving ourselves unconditionally. We literally birth aspects of ourselves that we have not learned to love out into the world through our children. Thus, our children always mirror back to us the parts of ourselves that we have not fully healed, loved, honored, respected, nurtured, integrated, accepted, forgiven, or expressed yet in our own lives. In other words our children bring to the surface all of our unresolved emotional pain, issues, and unmet needs from our own childhood. Fortunately, though, if you're a parent, through learning to love, respect, accept, appreciate, nurture, and forgive your children, you can in turn learn to love and heal all of yourself in the same way.

The same is also true for children. As children grow and develop they learn to master their love for themselves primarily through their relationships with their parents. Once again, if you have children yourself, then you're teaching your children to love themselves either through consciously embodying unconditional love yourself and encouraging them to do the same or, you're unconsciously challenging and strengthening their love for themselves by not loving them unconditionally. Either way, we all eventually learn the importance of loving, honoring, and valuing ourselves through this life-long intimate relationship.

As "adults", our own parents are often the people who influence us the most as we (1) form our relationship to ourselves and (2) create our lives over time. Thus the amount of love we have for ourselves in the present is strongly affected by the amount of love we feel toward our parents in the present. With this in mind, we cannot learn to love ourselves unconditionally if we cannot learn to love our parents unconditionally as well, ultimately because there is no separation between us and them.

For various reasons, this is one of the most challenging tasks that we're all called to accomplish in life, but it is indeed necessary both for the evolution of human consciousness and in mastering an unconditional love for ourselves. Through learning to love, accept, forgive, respect, and honor our parents unconditionally, we also master the necessary lessons to love ourselves and other people in the same ways. Thus, regardless of our current age, as the child of other human beings, we're constantly tested and challenged by our parents not only to love them unconditionally, but more importantly, to love ourselves unconditionally in relation to them. Hence, the evolutionary process by which we as human beings (1) move our genetic line forward and (2) awaken to the unconditional love that we are continues to unfold.

Over time, the universe expresses itself more fully with each new generation that is born. Through our own genes and our own biological families, God expresses another unique aspect of itself. This is another significant way that the universe loves itself through each and every one of us. In loving itself unconditionally, the universal self, or God's self, creatively expresses its divinity and beauty more fully through everyone and everything that comes to be. Through this process, God unfolds its greatest creative potential through each one of our individual lives. In other words, as we come to love ourselves unconditionally, we are in fact creating a life that is a unique expression of the universe's love for itself.

He who experiences the unity of life sees his own Self in all beings, and all beings in his own Self, and looks on everything with an impartial eye.

—BUDDHA

In awakening to the fact that all forms of love are indeed self-love, the voice of God within us guides us to *love all our human brothers, sisters, and neighbors in the same ways that we're all destined to love ourselves.* Through loving ourselves unconditionally we eventually develop a deep understanding and compassion for ourselves that naturally looks to understand and have compassion for all life, because deep inside we already know we're united with all that exists.

With this in mind, we live during a time where many of us still think, feel, act, and speak in ways that separate us from other human beings, ultimately because we've been conditioned to believe that our skin color, ethnic background, geographical location, religious faith, education, or economic status makes us different or separate from those who do not share the same beliefs, physical attributes, or lifestyle preferences that we do. The truth, however, is that there is nothing that separates us from anyone or anything besides the cocoon of our ego and the limiting beliefs and unprocessed emotions that make it up.

We've all just become attached to ideas about life that separate us from other people because we're scared of feeling the emotional pain that lives beneath the defensive and fragmented aspects of our personality. Almost every single one of us identifies with a limiting belief about who we are or what life is about, because this protects us from some form of suffering that's still unhealed within us. We become attached to limiting beliefs because we fear not knowing who we are if we (1) stop identifying with what we've been conditioned to believe by our parents, religion, or society, and (2) stop blindly believing what the people around us believe. We also fear the ultimate truth that we are actually one with all life and also one with God, because in accepting this we cannot blame, judge, or hate anyone or anything outside ourselves ever again. If we really are God in human form, then we're not only responsible for everything we've created and experienced throughout our own lives, but we're also responsible for everything that occurs within our world—which is a huge realization.

Hence, underneath our fears of accepting our unity with all life, we once again find emotional pain that we must transform and heal in order to embody our soul's enlightened true nature. As is true in every circumstance, through loving ourselves unconditionally we heal the pain that we fear and thereby break free of our unconscious needs for protection, judgment, and separation. Thankfully, as we intentionally transform our inner struggles, we not only let go of the fear-based, limiting beliefs that separate us from our true selves and from other people, but we also organically remember our unity with, and love for, all that exists.

CHAPTER TWENTY-FIVE

Self-Love Is the Road to Selflessness

Self-care is never a selfish act—it is simply good stewardship of the only gift I have, the gift I was put on earth to offer to others.

—PARKER PALMER

> *Wherever you are, please take a few slow, deep breaths into your belly. Please also feel your whole body, from your feet all the way up to the crown of your head, and then down to your fingertips. Please surrender fully and accept everything that you're thinking, feeling, and experiencing here in this moment. Please be present to your body and your breath.*

C ontrary to what many of us read or are led to believe, we must completely love the self that we have before we can ever consider losing it. To realize the enlightened state of consciousness that is often referred to as *selflessness*, each of us must first come to love our "self" unconditionally. Many of us on a spiritual path today aim to *lose ourselves* through spiritual practices, or through devoting ourselves to what we perceive to be selfless service, because culturally, spiritually, and religiously we've been taught that by helping others, as opposed to helping ourselves, we are living in an enlightened way. Living a life of service to humanity is undoubtedly an evolved way of life that we're all ultimately heading toward; however, too many of us unconsciously try to lose ourselves in other people's needs, desires, and problems before we've actually healed our own internal conflicts and unresolved emotional pain.

If we're honest with ourselves we'll see that many of us use spirituality and religion as a means to escape or avoid what's really going on in our own lives. In many cases we believe we're helping other people without self-interest when in reality we're unconsciously trying to lose ourselves in the desires, needs, and troubles of other people just so we don't have to look at ourselves or our own lives honestly. For many devoted parents, teachers, employees, health care practitioners, and religious followers, selfless service, martyrdom, or a fixation on selflessness, often becomes a means of denial and repression rather than a pure intention to help and serve other people.

In reaction to not loving all of who we are, many of us unconsciously try to lose ourselves and distract ourselves from the self, the past, and the life that we do not love. We often *try to be "selfless," "spiritual," "religious," "good," or "holy"* because deep down we're not at peace, happy, or satisfied, and we mistakenly believe that our inner battles will just go away if we simply divert ourselves from them.

Viewing ourselves from this perspective, it becomes very clear that selfishly cultivating unconditional love, kindness, and compassion for ourselves is the only way to meet the world and serve the world consciously and genuinely, essentially because we can only give what we actually have to give. If we do not have a conscious, kind, and self-aware relationship with ourselves that is based on unconditional love, then we cannot truly be loving, kind, and compassionate toward other people without resenting what we give or do for them.

When we unconsciously focus on other people's problems or needs in an attempt to avoid our own struggles we not only cause ourselves and the world more pain, but we also betray the purpose for which we were born. As we selfishly heal our psychological, emotional, and physical pain and thus grow in love for ourselves, however, we truly do become a pure source of selfless love in the world. As Mahatma Gandhi so beautifully expressed, "Be the change you wish to see in the world."

And the best way for each of us to be this change is to be selfish enough and brave enough to master loving ourselves unconditionally.

A person who seeks help for a friend, while
needy himself, will be answered first.

—THE TALMUD

When we live without love for ourselves, we always meet the world from a place of lack, inadequacy, and insecurity, no matter how well we mask it by our so-called selfless acts. From this place of denial we can never truly feel good about giving, because we always resent ourselves and others for giving what we do not truly have or want to give.

When we live with parts of ourselves, our lives, or our past that we have not fully embraced, there's no amount of selfless action that will ever offset or cancel out the unresolved guilt, shame, insecurity, anger, or hurt that we've stored in our body and which is now unconsciously driving our actions. Regardless of how many "good deeds" we do in the world, our soul will always call us back home to heal and love what we do not love within us so we can live in the world and give to the world from a place of purity, wholeness, and authenticity.

The truth is we can only help other people or help the world to the degree that we've already helped ourselves. And the only way to help ourselves is by loving ourselves enough to free ourselves from the psychological and emotional suffering that most of us prefer to deny and avoid. If we genuinely want to love and care for the world, each of us must (1) continually love and care for ourselves and (2) keep our own reserves not only full, but also full of pure intent. Thus, the most selfless and most challenging goal we can aim toward is to become a shining, enlightened example to others of true inner peace, health, happiness, and fulfillment, because in all honesty, what good are we to anyone if we're in pain, poor, starving, unhealthy, or miserable?

At some stage in our spiritual awakening it becomes crystal clear that loving ourselves unconditionally is the path to the enlightened state of consciousness that we term "selflessness," because as we liberate ourselves from our suffering, we transcend the constricting boundaries of our ego and we begin to experience our true self as being united with the universal self and with God. Eventually, our old ideas about who we are and what we are fall away, and our felt self-awareness finally expands to include everyone and everything that exists in the entire universe.

In terms of spiritual liberation, loving ourselves unconditionally is unquestionably the most direct path to enlightenment, because as we come to love ourselves at progressively deeper levels of our being, we shed the limiting beliefs that separate us from our true selves, from each other, and from all life, and thus liberate our soul. Simply through healing our psychological and emotional wounds here in the present moment, our perceived identity changes and expands until it eventually includes more magnificence, wisdom, and love than we could even begin to imagine.

Genuine selflessness naturally occurs when we're able to lose ourselves fully and purposefully in love, in the here and now, without avoiding pain or fear. Whether our love is directed toward ourselves, toward another human being, toward nature, toward the universe, or toward God, we eventually experience freedom from the confines of a separate self when our consciousness, attention, and energy are focused solely on whom and what we love.

However, in the same way that it is impossible to have selflessness in the world without also having selfishness, it is also impossible to have unconditional love in the world without having unconditional love for ourselves. These seemingly contradictory opposites not only define each other, they also exist purposefully to wake us up and to illuminate our ever-present wholeness. In fact, it's the mysterious space between these paradoxes that creates the most direct path to our psychological, emotional, physical, financial, and spiritual freedom.

CHAPTER TWENTY-SIX

Count Your Blessings
Every Day

*Gratefulness for what is there is one of the most powerful
tools for creating what is not yet there. What does gratefulness
mean? It means you appreciate what is. You value, you give
attention to, you honor whatever is here at this moment.*

—ECKHART TOLLE

*Wherever you are, please take a few slow, deep breaths into
your belly. Please also feel your whole body, from your feet all
the way up to the crown of your head, and then down to your
fingertips. Please surrender fully and accept everything that
you're thinking, feeling, and experiencing here in this moment.
Please be present to your body and your breath.*

L ife itself is the ultimate gift, yet most of us completely take it for
granted. Many of us become so trapped in negative thinking that
we constantly overlook all the aspects of our lives that we can appreciate
each day. By consciously looking for things to be grateful for, however,
even when we're struggling, we can find freedom from our suffering
immediately. In fact, the high vibrational energy of gratitude naturally
activates an enlightened awareness with which we both create and
attract positive experiences and situations. We often don't realize that

simply by appreciating the positive things *that are working in our lives right now*, even if they seem minimal, we'll always find that we have more and more to be grateful for. Expressing gratitude, therefore, is like a key that opens our heart and mind to possibilities that are unimaginable from a contracted and negative state of consciousness. And this is why creating intentional space each day to honor and appreciate all that we can in our lives is vital to finding lasting inner peace, health, happiness, and fulfillment.

Even when we're not feeling stuck or negative, many of us still become so caught up in our daily routines that we rarely take the time to reflect on and savor the numerous blessings in our lives. What most of us never learned is that creating space each day to express gratitude not only helps us to feel happy and content here in the present moment, but it also significantly enriches all of our positive life experiences as well.

Knowing this, the possibilities for expressing gratitude on a daily basis are truly infinite and never-ending. Aspects of our lives like our health, our home, food, clean water, the warmth of the sun's rays, any amount of money or financial support that we have, our past education, our teachers, our methods of transportation, our job, our family, our parents, our children, our partner or our spouse, our friends, our pets, the intelligent functions of our body, our mind, our cells, our organs, and our bones—all of these are blessings that we can learn to appreciate each and every day.

Simply cultivating gratitude for the life we've been given, for the opportunity to experience life and love as a human being, is the most powerful and most important place to start. In fact, if you stop right now, wherever you are, take a few slow, deep breaths into your belly, feel into your body, into the life that you are, and then look around with an open heart and mind, how can you truly not feel gratitude for the beauty, magic, and profundity of this life? If you *really look* at the trees, the birds, the sky, or the people around you, how can you not just sit back in awe? Life really is amazing, no matter how stuck we feel. We just have to teach ourselves to look for the magic in the mundane and for the light in the darkness, because they're both always present.

The best way to accomplish an improved environment is to focus upon the best things about where you currently are until you flood your own vibrational patterns of thought with appreciation; and in that changed vibration, you can allow the new-and-improved conditions and circumstances to come into your experience. Look for good things about where you are, and in your state of appreciation, you lift all self-imposed limitations (and all limitations are self-imposed) and free yourself for the receiving of wonderful things.

—ESTHER AND JERRY HICKS, THE TEACHINGS OF ABRAHAM

Thankfully, through cultivating unconditional love for ourselves, we naturally develop unconditional love and gratitude for our lives as well. We start to appreciate everything in life so much more, because when we do not place conditions on our own love for ourselves in the present, we do not place conditions on the love and appreciation we have for life either. In the same way we learn to love, accept, honor, and value ourselves independently of external conditions and circumstances, we also come to love, accept, honor, and value every single moment just the way it is.

Expressing gratitude, therefore, is one of the most important acts of self-love that we can engage in each day, because it frees us psychologically, emotionally, physically, financially, and spiritually more effectively than any other act or approach. Counting our blessings each day not only reflects the love and respect that we have for ourselves and our lives, but it also brings this love and respect out more fully into the world.

Thus, the more we give thanks for our lives, for the people in our lives, for all the little blessings in our lives, for all the blessings of the past, and even for all the blessings to come, the more fully we embody a deep love and appreciation for all that exists. Life already is such a numinous, wonder-filled experience that can be so joyful and so fulfilling if only we allow it to be. We just have to be brave enough to open our hearts completely right here in the present moment and allow the beauty, love, and blessings all around us to come pouring into and through our being. If we can find the courage, strength, and love for ourselves to do this, all that's left is to continue giving thanks for our lives, for the people in our lives, and for the infinite blessings that are always on their way.

A great deal of the chaos in the world occurs because
people don't appreciate themselves.

—CHOGYAM TRUNGPA RINPOCHE

Quite beautifully, the less we take for granted in life, the more we're granted access to everything we seek. When we take the time daily to acknowledge our life's many blessings, we not only fill our body, heart, and mind with more peace, health, happiness, and love, but we also ignite the energy within us that's necessary to do, experience, create, feel, and accomplish whatever we want to or need to. Hence, training our mind to (1) look for and (2) focus on the positive things around us is actually a key to creating what we want and need most in all aspects of our lives. The enlightened and nourishing energy of gratitude literally fulfills us while it simultaneously fuels our most valued intentions and goals, thereby providing us with the love for ourselves and for life necessary to create the high quality existence we all both desire and deserve.

It certainly is a very subtle dance between wanting and needing "more" in life while simultaneously cultivating acceptance and appreciation for everything just as it is. And this is precisely why taking time every day to ask ourselves what we're grateful for in and about our lives is so essential to being happy. Ultimately, counting our blessings on a daily basis is the one factor that balances the force inside each of us that is always driving our soul's evolution and expansion with the vital need in our heart to always be at peace and fulfilled in the here and now.

Heal Yourself Now Questions

Whom and what are you grateful for in your life right now?

What are all of the little things and the big things
that you can appreciate in and about your life?

*Contemplating these blessings each morning before you get out
of bed and every night before you fall asleep is one of the most
powerful spiritual and healing practices you can do for yourself.*

Whom and what are you grateful for from the past?

If you came across a genie right now and could ask for
anything you wanted or needed, what would you ask
for if there were no limits to what was possible?

(A)
Please make a detailed list with as many requests as you can think of.

(B)
Now, try imagining what life would *look like and feel like* if what you
desired already was your reality. Please feel it in your body and see
it in your mind. Please be as detailed as possible. Please try closing
your eyes and visualizing your desired reality for a few moments.

(C)
Then, please say, "Thank you, God (or universe) for (my
soul mate, health, happiness, car, money, adventure, new
job)," as though you already have what you asked for.

(D)
Try practicing this technique often. The more you do so, the
sooner you will attract your wishes and desires into your reality.

Love Yourself Now Affirmations

Thank you for my life. I am so blessed.

Thank you for my healthy body, mind, and heart.

Thank you for my healthy organs, bones, and cells.

Thank you for my family and friends.

Thank you for my mother and father.

Thank you for my partner.

Thank you for my children.

Thank you for the roof over my head.

Thank you for my bed.

Thank you for my job.

Thank you for nourishing food and clean water.

Thank you for the sunshine.

Thank you to the earth.

Thank you for the amazing years to come.

I am grateful to know that I have no idea
how amazing my life can be.

The more thankful I am, the more I have to be thankful for.

Thank you for today. Thank you for this moment.

CHAPTER TWENTY-SEVEN

Focus on Feeling
Alive and Well

Things are coming into your experience in response to your vibration.
Your vibration is offered because of the thoughts you are thinking, and you
can tell by the way you feel what kinds of thoughts you are thinking. Find
good-feeling thoughts, and good-feeling manifestations MUST follow. Make
a decision to look for the best feeling aspects of whatever you must give your
attention to, and otherwise look only for good-feeling things to give your
attention to- and your life will become one of increasingly good-feeling aspects.

—ESTHER AND JERRY HICKS, THE TEACHINGS OF ABRAHAM

Wherever you are, please take a few slow, deep breaths into
your belly. Please also feel your whole body, from your feet all
the way up to the crown of your head, and then down to your
fingertips. Please surrender fully and accept everything that
you're thinking, feeling, and experiencing here in this moment.
Please be present to your body and your breath.

E ach day we are faced with decisions in our personal and professional
lives that ultimately shape the course of our destiny and the quality
of our health, our happiness, our relationships and our daily experience
of life. If we want to live our lives to the fullest, be well, and respect
ourselves for the life we've created, it is crucial that we each master

making choices that are aligned with who we truly are, why we're really here, and how we genuinely feel.

A simple but powerful way to achieve this is to look at each moment as a fork in the road on the path to our most liberated, joyful and authentic life. In any given scenario, at least one direction will always represent a decision that does not feel good in our heart or in our body. In this same situation at least one other direction or path will eventually reveal itself, which represents a decision that undoubtedly feels very good and exciting in our heart and in our body.

Quite often it can be confusing as to which path is best or healthiest for us to choose. It's very common to feel unclear about which decision feels good and which does not. In situations like this it is best to wait, or not make any major choices until a clear knowing surfaces from deep within us. Although this seems like common sense, many of us struggle on a daily basis to know and act on what feels optimal for us.

The primary reason for this is that our thoughts are often at odds with what we feel in our hearts, because our minds have become very good at trying to protect our hearts from emotional pain. This dynamic leads most of us to feel as though our heads and our hearts are pointing us in opposite directions, when in reality they are both simply guiding us home to ourselves—to our inner truth—here in the present moment.

Because many of us have become so cut off from what we instinctually feel in our heart, we now live trapped in our head, running in mental circles overanalyzing important decisions. Thankfully this mental confusion is merely a symptom that's guiding us deeper into what we *feel in our body*, so we can finally heal the repressed emotional pain that stops our heart and mind from feeling united and in agreement.

Another very important point to understand is that our new direction forward, or the next step, will not become clear until we've fully learned the lessons we're meant to master in the current situation. We will often stay in something that does not feel good or healthy until we learn to love and value ourselves enough to only enter into situations and relationships that support us to feel well and free. In other words we unconsciously stay in situations that do not feel good until we learn to fully express what we feel, stick up for ourselves, and find clarity around what we actually do want.

In my experience, a YES-WORTHY direction will always reveal itself when we're truly ready to take the next step. Once we have processed all of the emotions and lessons that are present in the current circumstances, the best path forward will become illuminated by positive feelings and clear thoughts that make us feel so good we cannot deny the direction life is now guiding us to explore.

While waiting for our next step to become well-defined, besides simply identifying what we're feeling, wanting and needing right now, the most effective thing we can focus our time and energy on is doing the small things in life that make us feel good, alive and well. Whether this is taking short walks, writing, reading, taking a bath, making ourselves something warm to drink, exercising, listening to music, painting, or having fun with genuine people, by concentrating on what makes us feel good in the here and now, we can enjoy our lives in the present more deeply—while we simultaneously distinguish where and with whom we currently do not feel good, or where and with whom we do not love ourselves enough to honor the very best we're capable of creating.

What activities, small or large, make you feel good, alive and well?

What activities make you feel happy or bring out joy inside of you?

Which people or environments do you feel great around, simply because you can be yourself, or explore yourself, or do what feels true and healthy for you?

By identifying your answers to these questions and then by focusing on these activities and relationships as much as possible each day, you will begin to increase the amount of time you feel good, alive and well overall. With consistency this process will bring significant clarity to larger life decisions, goals, and plans because the more you focus your energy on simply feeling good, the more you will naturally feel and know which choices are most aligned with who you really are, why you're really here, and the quality of life you'd like to create.

Because the purpose of human life is to enjoy it fully, while learning what it means to love unconditionally, filling our days with the small things that make us feel great is vital to creating the harmonious and fulfilling life we all dream of. The small daily choices that build our energy, mood, and health, as opposed to those that drain our energy or bring us down, are what provide us with the fuel we need to make our larger visions, goals, and desires our lived reality.

Without focusing on the small things that make us feel good on a daily basis, we cannot access the energy we need to move forward in creating a life that reflects the greatness we're all capable of. Regardless of how attractive a certain lifestyle, career, relationship, or dream-reality is, we will never create it without acting in ways that make us feel better and better each day. Wanting something strongly is not enough to make it so. We have to love, honor, and authentically express ourselves each day so we have the energy to do what needs to be done, to get us where we ultimately want to be.

Coming full circle, each and every moment is a junction on our path to liberation—to lasting inner peace, health, happiness and fulfillment. YES-WORTHY opportunities will always present themselves to us, especially when we're focused on what makes us feel alive and well. If we can learn to act when it feels good, but wait to act when it does not feel good, our heart will always guide us toward the lasting love, joy, and peace we're seeking.

CHAPTER TWENTY-EIGHT

Cultivate Your Inner Wealth

*Let us more and more insist on raising funds of love, of
kindness, of understanding, of peace. Money will come if we
seek first the Kingdom of God—the rest will be given.*

—MOTHER TERESA

*Wherever you are, please take a few slow, deep breaths into
your belly. Please also feel your whole body, from your feet all
the way up to the crown of your head, and then down to your
fingertips. Please surrender fully and accept everything that
you're thinking, feeling, and experiencing here in this moment.
Please be present to your body and your breath.*

Each of us holds different beliefs about what constitutes true wealth
and true success in life. However, anyone who has chased after
money, material wealth, or worldly success as a top priority at the
expense of their health, their relationships, or their inner states of peace,
happiness, or fulfillment deeply knows that true wealth and true success
are not measured by the amount of money we have in the bank or by
the material possessions we own.

In today's world, many of us have been raised to think of success
primarily in terms of attaining financial wealth and material abundance,
but again, these achievements mean nothing if we do not have love for

195

ourselves, love for our lives, and love for the people in our lives. If we're not completely happy and at peace within ourselves, our relationships, and our careers, even if we have both fame and fortune, just how wealthy and successful are we, really?

Inevitably, there always comes a time when we realize that true wealth and true success come in the forms of unconditional love, inner peace, health, happiness, connection, and deep fulfillment. When we have love in our lives each day, love in our heart, love in our relationships, and love in our work, then and only then are we living a truly wealthy and successful life. When we're at peace, healthy, happy, and fulfilled, we've cultivated a type of inner success and wealth that nothing and no one can ever take away from us—a form of lived prosperity that nothing could ever truly compare to.

Deep down we all want to live each day feeling that our lives express our innermost truths, values, and dreams, because we know this is what demonstrates a genuinely successful and wealthy life. We all want to wake up each morning with clarity about who we are and passion for why we are here, because we know that finding this ever-present source of inner wealth unlocks a type of courage, confidence, and integrity that no amount of money could ever create or buy.

For what is a man profited, if he shall gain the
whole world, and lose his own soul?

—MATTHEW 16:26

For those of us who struggle to create financial freedom it is crucial to understand that it is the depth of our inner wealth and success that determines the degree to which we create lasting wealth and success in the outer world. As much as we've all been led to believe otherwise, accumulating material wealth or security before we attend to our inner wealth will only result in unhappiness and dissatisfaction. Even though we tend to think that money and worldly success are the key ingredients in living a healthy, happy, and fulfilling life, on a deeper level, we all know that these things will never satisfy our inner hunger for clarity of purpose, heart-to-heart connection, and true self-respect. Thus, as odd as it may seem at first, loving ourselves unconditionally is not only the key to transforming our suffering and fulfilling our life's purpose, but it is also a very effective way to create sustainable external wealth, success, and financial freedom as well.

For those of us who have already created financial freedom, but who are now looking for true love, peace, health, happiness, fulfillment, or deeper meaning in life, the previous chapters in this book offer you the keys to creating a type of wealth that no amount of money or external achievement could ever purchase. Considering this, if you've already created financial wealth in your life, it is important to ask yourself: *why? Where did your motivations come from? Were you conditioned to make money by your family and society? Were you seeking love, approval, attention, or praise? Were you afraid for your survival or the survival of your family? Did you accumulate material wealth out of what you believed was necessity? Did you believe that money and material wealth would make you more loveable, attractive, emotionally secure, or happy? Did you believe money would give you power, influence, or control?*

Regardless of your answers to these questions, the fact remains that loving ourselves unconditionally, while also finding deep purpose and connection in our lives, is the key to discovering the inner wealth that (1) we all desire and (2) is ultimately already ours.

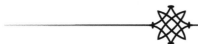

On the healing and spiritual journey, it's easy to become trapped in the idea that one must renounce or reject money or the material world in order to find lasting peace, health, happiness, or fulfillment. But when we stop to consider that everything in the universe is unquestionably a part of God, it becomes clear that there's no true separation between what is "spiritual" and what is "material." Thus, when we reject the material world, for any reason, we're merely denying a very large part of ourselves that we must eventually embrace. Likewise, however, if we do not honor our soul's deeper inner calling, we're just abandoning both who we are and why we are here—until of course the universe forces us to our knees in surrender.

If we truly want freedom from our suffering, we eventually have to value and respect both the inner and the outer aspects of our lives. At the same time, we must also remember that money and material possessions will never make us more loveable, more worthy, more deserving, more happy, more connected, or more emotionally secure. Intuitively, we already know that our inner truths must take priority over any form of external wealth, achievement, gain, or recognition. Even though we temporarily forget this, deep in our soul we all know we must master loving ourselves unconditionally so we can (1) fulfill our life's purpose and (2) bring genuine peace, love, and happiness into this world.

Although many of us have closed our heart and mind to making money or creating material wealth, money itself is not bad in any way. *It is our relationship to money that is either healthy or not.* In fact, money is just another form of energy, or love. If our happiness and sense of self-worth are based on how much money or material wealth we have, then our relationship to money is both unhealthy and limiting. However, if we know that money cannot buy happiness or love, and that we must love ourselves and answer our inner calling as a top priority, then our relationship to money can be both healthy and liberating.

The same logic also applies to the material world of "things" or "possessions." Things and possessions are not bad in and of themselves. There is nothing wrong or sinful about enjoying beautiful clothing, homes, cars, or other material possessions. Just like money, it is our inner relationship to material objects (or lack there of) that is either healthy or unhealthy. If we believe that material possessions will make us more loveable, worthy, deserving, happy, or less insecure, then our relationship to the "things" we either have or desire is definitely unhealthy. Likewise, if we identify with our material possessions and thus believe they (1) somehow define us or (2) make us superior or inferior to others in any way, then again our relationship to these material objects will always cause us to suffer.

Conversely, when we prioritize our inner wealth—our inner peace, health, happiness, fulfillment, and love for ourselves—we can enjoy the physical world without being attached to anything. If we know that "things" will never bring us happiness, deep meaning, or true love, we can create and experience all forms of material wealth without losing ourselves or deluding ourselves into thinking we will ever find what we're looking for outside ourselves.

> *To live content with small means; to seek elegance rather than luxury, and refinement rather than fashion; to be worthy, not respectable, and wealthy, not, rich; to listen to stars and birds, babes and sages, with an open heart; to study hard; to think quietly, act frankly, talk gently, await occasions, hurry never; in a word, to let the spiritual, unbidden and unconscious, grow up through the common. This is my symphony.*

—WILLIAM ELLERY CHANNING

Whether we'd like to create greater financial freedom or, we'd simply like to find a more fulfilling approach to making money, we're all being called to open our minds and accept a new way of thinking about money and, in particular, its direct relationship to love. Practically speaking, it is crucial that we come to understand the intimate relationship between (1) how much we love ourselves, (2) how much love we give to others, (3) how open and vulnerable our hearts are, and (4) how wealthy and successful we are externally. In other words, if we truly want to thrive in today's evolving world, we actually have no choice but to master the intimate dynamic that's always unfolding between money, love, and the energetic structure of our universe.

At this point in human evolution it's critical we all realize that everything in the universe is made of one fundamental energetic substance, which permeates all life and also drives the function and movement of all life in its various forms. Practically speaking, both love and money can be viewed simply as different manifestations of the same basic energy that makes up everything that exists. Thus, beneath the apparent differences between our body, our thoughts, money, material objects, and the state of being that we call love, there is one underlying, uniting force or tapestry—which is the intelligent, logical, aware, and energetic universe.

You might be wondering, *Why is this important to understand in terms of living a wealthy, successful, and financially liberated life?*

The reason why these insights are so important and so empowering is that while there are many ways to make money and create material wealth in the short term, *there is only one way to manifest sustainable, long-term financial abundance and live a successful, fulfilling life that is aligned with the universe, with our life's purpose, and with who we truly are.*

This one way is always through following our heart's inner guidance and through living with our heart completely open and vulnerable, because when we live openheartedly we allow the infinite source of love and energy that's both within us and all around us to pour into, from, and through our being. Even though you might be skeptical at first, the truth remains that it's only through continuously expanding our heart's capacity to give and receive love that we can open ourselves to the unlimited stream of universal wealth-love-energy that is always available to us.

Here in the present moment, the only obstacles that block us from unlimited internal and external wealth are (1) our limiting beliefs around needing to be more, do more, or have more to finally be loveable or happy and (2) our unhealed emotional pain. Beyond these limiting beliefs and unhealed emotions, our true nature is, has been, and always will be an infinite source of all that we could ever want or need to live wealthy, successful, and abundant lives.

Even though we've never learned how wealthy we all naturally are, it doesn't change the fact that each of us is united with the infinite, abundant, and limitless consciousness that is God, the universe, or the source of all that is. Thus, our beliefs and feelings around being lacking or inadequate in any way only exist to (1) help us remember the universe's higher logic, or rationale, and (2) master the science of creating wealth, success, and freedom both internally and externally.

As we've seen before, we all create our lives as we experience them in the outer world based upon the subtle energies of our beliefs, thoughts, emotions, actions, and spoken words. If we explore this process of creation on an even deeper level, we'll naturally see that our beliefs, thoughts, and emotions ultimately drive the actions that we take and the words that we speak. From this perspective, it becomes quite clear that the more consistently our beliefs, thoughts, and emotions come from a place of inner wealth, success, and abundance—in other words, from a place of unconditional self-love—then the more our actions and spoken words will come from an energy of wealth, success, and abundance as well. It logically follows that the more often our beliefs, thoughts, emotions, actions, and spoken words all come from an energy and consciousness of inner wealth, success, and abundance, or once again from a place of unconditional self-love, then the more our lives in the outer world will reflect back to us this inner, soul-based prosperity.

When we truly love, honor, value, and respect ourselves, we organically create wealthy, successful, and abundant situations, both personally and professionally, because wealth, success, and abundance are merely the natural byproducts of a healthy relationship with ourselves. The more love we give to and have for ourselves, the more we fill ourselves up with loving, positive energy—with health, happiness, peace, passion, and fulfillment—and this process always translates into natural feelings of inner wealth, success, and abundance. Thus, the more we feel wealthy, successful, and abundant internally, the more energy and love we have to give to every person and situation in our lives.

On top of this, when we make conscious choices each day to honor both ourselves and our life's purpose, we're living in a way that's constantly fulfilling our reserves, which always results in natural and consistent forms of generosity. When we create our days from a place of deep love and respect for ourselves, we literally fill our body, heart, and mind to the point where we're overflowing with positive, loving energy, and, in the same way a rose cannot help but give out its fragrance, we cannot help but effortlessly give out what is bursting forth from within.

It doesn't matter what form the passionate, purposeful sharing of our inner wealth takes, because we always receive back the energy we give out in the forms we need most at any particular point in our lives. It might be money, food, shelter, work, companionship, external recognition, or some other form of external fulfillment. Regardless of what comes back to us, we always receive exactly what we need when we're committed to bringing forth our inner wealth fully into the world.

Ultimately, by cultivating our inner wealth the overflowing abundance within us cannot help but come back to us as abundant wealth in the outer world. This is the case because the more we love ourselves, the more we're able to love other people as well; and the more we're able to love ourselves and others, the more open and vulnerable our hearts become; and the more open and vulnerable our hearts become, the more we're able to give and receive love in its various forms (i.e. money, compassion, presence, energy). So, as mind-boggling as it may seem, the amount of money, material wealth, and worldly success that we experience, or in other words, the amount of energy and love that we receive back from life, is directly proportional to (1) how open our hearts are and (2) the amount of love we're willing to give to ourselves and to the world. Even though our relationships to money tend to be quite complicated, confusing, and stressful, living prosperously really is quite simple once we view it in this light.

For true love is inexhaustible; the more you give, the more you have. And if you go to draw at the true fountainhead, the more water you draw, the more abundant is its flow.

—Antoine de Saint-Exupery

Although you may not hear this often enough, you are undoubtedly capable of creating the financial freedom you desire in life. Whether or not you end up experiencing this freedom all depends on how much responsibility you're willing to take for the amount of love, acceptance, value, and respect you cultivate for yourself, your life, and your life's purpose.

Our individual capacities to create financial freedom and material wealth are unlimited. However, most of us don't actually need that much money to be happy. We just need enough to take care of our responsibilities while we fulfill our life's purpose and enjoy our lives as much as possible each day. Deep down we all know that money can't buy the most valuable things in life. So even if we had all the money in the world, we could not purchase the heart-to-heart connections, peace, happiness, or love that we all want and need.

If your relationship to money currently causes you to suffer, your soul is asking you to accept that you can only create external wealth to the degree that you love, honor, respect, and value both yourself and your destined work in the world. Thus, you are being called to define what personally represents "the good life," or a liberated life, so you can intentionally focus on creating it with awareness and personal responsibility.

Fortunately, when we follow our heart and go after what we sincerely desire, we'll always create exactly what we need to support our lifestyle and way of being in the world. When we're focused on fulfilling our soul's purpose, the universe and God always provide us with everything we need to (1) enjoy our lives to the fullest and (2) be at peace. For one person this could be twenty thousand dollars per year, and for another person it may be one hundred thousand or even one million dollars per year. Regardless, it's ultimately a waste of time and energy to judge another person based on how much money they make or what they have. All we can do is focus on valuing, honoring, and loving ourselves enough to create what we personally desire, dream of, and deserve.

Thankfully, we live in an infinite universe, so there's always enough to go around. The mere fact that one person has a large amount of happiness, love, money, or success, does not mean there's not enough for us to fulfill our own unique potential and live each day to the fullest. Life merely asks each of us to find enough patience to cultivate the inner wealth and success that always precede the sustainable external wealth and long-term success that we were all born to experience.

Since we're not only one hundred percent responsible for what we create, but also one hundred percent capable of creating anything we truly want, it's entirely up to us to persist in breaking through the inner blocks that are stopping us from (1) loving ourselves unconditionally, (2) opening our hearts completely, (3) accepting our life's inherent worth, and (4) finding the inner peace, health, happiness, and fulfillment that always lead to unlimited wealth and success in all forms. In the end, there are no words to describe the high quality prosperity and aliveness that are born from loving ourselves unconditionally and fulfilling our life's destined purpose.

Heal Yourself Now Questions

What do wealth and success mean to you?

What will your life look like when you feel wealthy and successful?

If you had all the money you desired right now,
what would you go do, create, or experience?

Do you actually need more money to do, create,
and experience *all* of these things?

Do you feel that your heart is fully open? Do you feel
that you love life and people with your whole heart?
If not, why not? When will you take the risk and give
all of yourself to your life and your purpose?

Are you professionally engaged in work that you love?

If not, when will you stop compromising yourself?

Do you overspend or compulsively spend money?

*If so, can you see that the reason you do this is because you're still not
accepting yourself fully? Can you see how spending money numbs you
temporarily to certain things within yourself and your life? Can you see
how underneath this habit there are things about you, your life, and
your past that you still do not love, accept, forgive, or feel good about?
Can you see how the root cause of your overspending is connected to
where in your life you're compromising, abandoning, betraying, and
thus hurting yourself? Can you see that regardless of what you buy your
insecurities do not go away? Can you see how subconsciously you believe*

that having more, or buying more, will make you more loveable, more attractive, or more secure in yourself? Can you see how this is connected to the conditional love, acceptance, and approval you seek from others?

Are you afraid of spending money?

If so, can you see how this relates to you being afraid of feeling vulnerable? Can you see that you fear feeling the insecurity and inadequacy within you and thus try to cover them by hoarding money or material possessions? Are you aware of your fears around giving and receiving love? Can you see how you fear being abandoned, betrayed, used, or hurt, and thus feel the need to hold back and over control yourself and your true desires? Can you see how underneath your fear of "not having enough," you're really afraid of accepting and expressing what you truly feel, want, and need for yourself? Can you also see that you do not have complete trust in life because you do not trust yourself?

Love Yourself Now Affirmations

There is an infinite source of wealth within
me. My soul is eternally wealthy.

Self-love and self-respect are my path to true wealth and success.

Money will never buy me true love or happiness.

I am secure in myself with or without money.

Mother earth, God, and the universe always support me.

I love and accept myself just as I am. I am loveable just the way I am.

No amount of money can make me more loveable than I already am.

I deserve true love just as I am.

I deserve the financial freedom to live a joyful life that I love.

I have everything I need to create a wealthy,
successful, and fulfilling life.

Loving myself is the path to financial fulfillment and freedom.

The more I love myself, the more wealthy and successful I am.

My health and happiness are more valuable than money.

CHAPTER TWENTY-NINE

Take the Vulnerable Path

Leap and the net will appear.

—JOHN BURROUGHS

> *Wherever you are, please take a few slow, deep breaths into your belly. Please also feel your whole body, from your feet all the way up to the crown of your head, and then down to your fingertips. Please surrender fully and accept everything that you're thinking, feeling, and experiencing here in this moment. Please be present to your body and your breath.*

O ne of the most important realizations I've ever had in my own life is that it is not until we jump, take a leap of faith, and risk everything we've known before, that life can give us what we truly desire most. The logic behind this fact is that when we allow ourselves to be the victim of our fears—meaning we allow our fears of failure, judgment, pain, rejection, or the unknown to stop us from going confidently after what we want and dream of—our hearts remain closed, which literally blocks us from receiving the very things we've been seeking. In other words, when we allow our fears to drive our choices, *the actions we do not take* and *the opportunities we allow to pass us by* are symbolic of us rejecting the life we genuinely desire.

Conversely, when we find the courage to face our fears directly, to go after what we want and dream of, and thus jump into the unfamiliar territories that are calling out to us, our hearts literally open, which then renders us ready to finally receive what we've been waiting and longing to feel, achieve and experience. Once we finally love and value ourselves enough to trust the promises that life is continually whispering into our ears, it is time for us to take the risk, to step out beyond the cold-comfort that we know we're not satisfied with, and to open our hearts to the high quality life we've always been destined to live.

It is not the critic who counts; not the man who points out how the strong man stumbles, or where the doer of deeds could have done them better. The credit belongs to the man who is actually in the arena, whose face is marred by dust and sweat and blood; who strives valiantly; who errs, who comes short again and again, because there is no effort without error and shortcoming; but who does actually strive to do the deeds; who knows great enthusiasms, the great devotions; who spends himself in a worthy cause; who at the best knows in the end the triumph of high achievement, and who at the worst, if he fails, at least fails while daring greatly, so that his place shall never be with those cold and timid souls who neither know victory nor defeat.

—THEODORE ROOSEVELT

Authentic long-term success, whether it's in life, love, business, health, or spiritual awakening, is the direct result of our commitment to remain openhearted and vulnerable. In my experience, all successful endeavors—whether the goal is to love myself unconditionally, to fulfill my life's purpose, to build a thriving business, to express my attraction to a woman, to create a healthy relationship, or to find inner peace and freedom—each one boils down to my willingness to overcome rejection and the fear of being rejected. In other words, I have found that it is the persistence to continually jump, to push the edge of my comfort zone, to wear my heart on my sleeve, to express the truth in my heart, and to continually go after all I want and dream of—no matter what—that opens the door to my deepest desires in life.

Through courageously facing both rejection and the fear of rejection head on we eventually learn not to fear them, because the self-respect and self-confidence that come from being true to ourselves—from not holding ourselves back—is more valuable than a false sense of pride or security. At some point it becomes apparent that the pain we create by rejecting ourselves is far greater and far more destructive than any pain we could ever experience from being rejected or criticized by someone else for any reason. Once we finally understand this high truth, both the possibility of rejection and the fear of rejection lose their power over us, which then enables us to live vulnerably and to bravely jump whenever life calls us into the new or the unknown.

CHAPTER THIRTY

Never Settle for Less

All men dream: but not equally. Those who dream by night in the dusty recesses of their minds wake in the day to find that it was only vanity: but the dreamers of the day are dangerous men, for they may act on their dreams with open eyes and make them their reality.

—THOMAS E. LAWRENCE

> **Wherever you are, please take a few slow, deep breaths into your belly. Please also feel your whole body, from your feet all the way up to the crown of your head, and then down to your fingertips. Please surrender fully and accept everything that you're thinking, feeling, and experiencing here in this moment. Please be present to your body and your breath.**

In the same way that we were not born to suffer, we did not come here to settle for a half-lived life. Thus to truly be at peace, healthy, happy, and fulfilled within ourselves and our lives, each of us is called to take our love for ourselves to the deepest level of our being. As and when we do this, we activate latent potentials that live dormant in the depths of our soul, which, once ignited, empower us to make the choices and take the steps necessary to create our most liberated and joyful life.

In order to fulfill our life's purpose, we're all called to consciously create a life that reflects a unique, free, and full expression of who and what we truly are. In other words, as our love for ourselves truly becomes unconditional and full, the next step in our self-mastery and personal evolution is always the realization of our greatest potential.

If we were to name a final destination in this experience that we call life, it is one where we truly embody the infinite source of unconditional love alive within us. Our greatest calling is to lose ourselves fully in the ocean of love that we are so we may embody and share this love in all that we do.

As we master loving ourselves unconditionally, we simultaneously realize that our moment-to-moment choices are either leading us toward our ultimate goals in life or they're not. We're either honoring ourselves in every moment, situation, and relationship and therefore fulfilling our life's purpose or, we're denying our soul's deepest inner calling. Thus, self-mastery based on unconditional self-love requires us to channel the energies of our beliefs, thoughts, emotions, actions, and spoken words toward creating, achieving, doing, and experiencing all that our heart and soul are guiding us to do.

With this in mind, anytime that we set a conscious intention, or goal, it always brings into our awareness and experience all of the unconscious aspects of ourselves, our lives, and our past that need to be healed, let go of, or loved in order for us to reach the goal we've intuitively set for ourselves. In other words, all of the ways in which we compromise ourselves or sabotage ourselves from doing and achieving what we intend or desire must be recognized, faced, and broken through.

When we set any kind of intention, especially one to love ourselves unconditionally and free ourselves from our suffering, all of the limiting beliefs and unhealed emotions that are holding us back arise within us organically so we can transform them and let them go. Similarly, all of the unconscious ways in which we speak and act surface into our awareness so we can redirect our vital life force energies toward manifesting our ultimate intentions, visions, and dreams. Furthermore, every external situation and relationship that is not healthy or that does not reflect our purpose in life is naturally called into question because it either needs to be let go of completely or be completely transformed.

We are what we repeatedly do. Excellence, then, is not an act, but a habit.

—ARISTOTLE

Creating a life that truly reflects our greatest potential demands that we hold a conscious intention within our heart and mind not to settle for anything less than we're worthy, deserving, or capable of in any aspect of our lives. In loving ourselves unconditionally an inner resolve naturally emerges that cannot and will not settle for anything less than the joy, abundance, passion, and freedom that come when our lives truly demonstrate our inherent greatness.

Knowing this, what we focus our attention on in life is what we get, whether we consciously want it or not. So along with the intention to realize our greatest potential comes the task of deliberately focusing all our attention on the manifestation of it. Consciously creating a life that is deeply aligned with our heart and extremely liberating for our soul does not happen by chance. It happens because we intentionally focus on creating it with every choice we make and every breath we take.

Deep in our hearts we all know that to live each day with unconditional love, compassion, and kindness for ourselves and to express the beauty and wisdom inherent to our soul's true nature, is a life that brings the lasting happiness and profound fulfillment we're all looking for. To live each day abundantly and vibrantly in such a way that we feel interconnected with all life, at one with the entire universe, and at home in God is a life that truly reflects the purpose for which we were born.

The inner success and wealth that we all desire can only become our reality as we love ourselves and thus fill ourselves with the health, peace, and joy that are more valuable than any form of external achievement, material gain, or recognition. When we know without doubt that we've done and are doing all that we can each day to live our lives to the fullest, with intention, purpose, and awareness, we know our destiny is our reality and our liberation is here. When every belief, thought, emotion, action, and spoken word born within us is grounded in unconditional love for ourselves, other people, and all life, then we know with certainty that we have mastered unconditional self-love.

The evolutionary force of the universe is always driving the love within us to heal us and fulfill us completely from the inside out. Like a river that eventually flows back into the vast ocean, so too are we always being led home to the source of love, freedom, and infinite possibility from which we come. Just like caterpillars that have no choice but to become butterflies, you and I ultimately have no choice but to bring the love that we are fully into this world.

It's merely a matter of time.

Every single one of us is destined to liberate ourselves from our suffering, fulfill our life's purpose, and realize our greatest potential both personally and professionally, but we must know this, claim this, and wholeheartedly commit to bringing it forth. Please don't set yourself up for a life of regret that's full of I-could-haves or I-should-haves. Please love yourself enough now to break free into the bliss and joy that are your birthright. Please go after what you want and love in life and never settle for less than you know you are capable of.

Above all else, please never settle for a relationship with yourself or anyone else that is not based on and full of the unconditional love, kindness, and respect that you deserve. You were not born to suffer, so if you've truly had enough sickness, misery, and unhealthy compromise, you can and will heal yourself while you simultaneously create the magnificent, awakened, and self-actualized life you have always been destined to live.

Heal Yourself Now Questions

If you knew that you would die one year from today, what would you focus your time and energy on? What would you go do, see, and experience? Who would you call or reconnect with? Who would you forgive? Who would you spend more quality time with?

What does your most liberated and joyful life look like? What do you imagine the life of your dreams to feel like?

What steps do you know you need to take in order to make your larger vision and dream your reality? Why are you avoiding these steps? When will you stop making excuses and finally go after what you believe in, value, want, and love?

Where in your life are you settling for less than you know you are capable of?

Where and with whom in your life are you still compromising yourself and denying your greatness?

Once again, are you waiting for your children to age, your parents to die, or your intimate relationship to end before you start living your life the way you want to? If so, why?

When is enough truly enough? When will you say enough settling, enough compromising, enough sickness, enough misery, and enough living in fear?

If not now, then when? If not today, then when?

Love Yourself Now Affirmations

I was not born to suffer. I was born to live my life to the fullest.

I deserve the best in every aspect of my life.

I deserve to be happy.

It's never too late to start over. I can recreate anything I need to.

I am always supported and protected.

I will not settle for less than I am worthy, deserving, or capable of.

I have everything I need within me to
create a fulfilling life that I love.

CHAPTER THIRTY-ONE

The Final Question

There are only two mistakes one can make along the road
to truth; not going all the way, and not starting.

—Buddha

After many years of searching for the inner healing, purpose, and freedom that I believe we're all looking for in life, I began to ask myself:

If we truly are God in human form, and if we both chose and created our lives and all of our experiences in their entirety, in this lifetime as well as in all of our previous lifetimes, then why would we ever choose to suffer or create pain for ourselves or others? In other words, why would we ever choose to hurt ourselves by not loving ourselves? Why would we ever choose to forget who we truly are or why we came here? Why would we create an ego, or a separate self, and thereby forget our unity with God, the universe, and all life? Why would we choose to forget that our soul's true nature is an infinite source of pure, unconditional love and that we do not need to search for love outside of ourselves?

I asked myself these questions regularly for a period of time, because they felt like the final piece to the puzzle in our universal quest for lasting inner peace, health, happiness, fulfillment, and freedom. Eventually you could say I was shown, or that I remembered, that the sole reason why we all choose to forget who we truly are and thus create suffering for ourselves is so we may bring unconditional love fully into the physical world.

The logic behind this ultimate spiritual truth is that through learning to forgive ourselves fully for the pain and suffering we chose to create, we truly come to accept and love ourselves unconditionally, and this process is specifically designed to bring forth our capacity to accept and forgive other people, which is the essence of unconditional love.

The reason why this awareness is so important is that if we truly want to enjoy our lives—or, in other words, heal ourselves, fulfill our life's purpose, and awaken spiritually—we have no choice but to take full responsibility for *everything that we experience*. This means we cannot blame God, our parents, our children, our spouse, or anyone for any reason, because when we do, we just give away our personal power, health, happiness, and freedom. The only way to free ourselves from our suffering and thus create peace on this planet is to forgive both ourselves and others and then accept our unity with God, the universe, and all life.

In the beginning of my own healing and spiritual journey I believed that responsibility and freedom could not exist together. However, I later realized that in order to liberate myself from suffering and truly enjoy my life, I had to (1) commit fully to my life's purpose every day and (2) take complete responsibility for every single thought, emotion, and experience in my life.

Today, it is through a wholehearted devotion to loving myself unconditionally that life continually opens doors to an ever-expanding freedom, joy, and peace. With each new day I remember the agreements I made before this lifetime more clearly, and in these memories I find the strength and discipline to walk my destined path to the end, knowing that giving up or turning around are not options and will only lead to suffering.

DEPARTING WORDS

The one who follows the crowd will usually get no further than the crowd. The one who walks alone is likely to find himself in places no one has ever been.

—ALBERT EINSTEIN

As we've explored throughout this book, most of us were never taught growing up that we were not born to suffer. We also never learned that each of us has a purpose in this life and that through finding it and fulfilling it we would also discover lasting inner peace and happiness. Instead, the larger majority of us grew up watching our parents, our extended family members, and our role models struggle within themselves, their relationships, and their careers. In fact, many of us watched the "adults" in our lives battle day in and day out with addictions, anger, fear, depression, and regret while simultaneously trying to raise families, put food on the table, and find a breath of peace and happiness for themselves. The sad but purposeful truth is that our parents and most people alive today were never taught how to love themselves unconditionally or why it's so important to master as early as possible in life. As a result, our parents and the other adults who influenced us as children could not show us or teach us what they themselves were still struggling to learn. They couldn't help us to transform our own suffering, because they were still trying to find peace, health, happiness, and fulfillment within their own body, heart, and mind. They also couldn't meet our own need for love completely because they were often too busy seeking the love they needed for themselves.

Looking back on life from this perspective, it's easy to see how for generations people all over the world have struggled to master living in ways that are deeply joyful, harmonious, and satisfying. This is why the desire for freedom from our suffering has always surfaced organically from deep within the human heart. In the end, the desires for peace, health, happiness, and fulfillment always hold the highest value once the dust storms of fear, hatred, vanity, and materialism settle and give way to the clarity and light of unconditional love, kindness, and mutual respect.

Thus, regardless of our age or stage in life, when we look back on our own lives and we consider the hand of cards *we both chose and played over time*, it's hard not to feel compassion for ourselves and for the people closest to us. Likewise, when we really stop to reflect on the challenging lessons life presents to everyone in unique yet equal forms, it's difficult not to feel sympathy for our planet, for our ancestors, and for the generations to come.

As human beings we all struggle and yet we still find countless ways to judge ourselves and become insecure for feeling the way we feel, for creating the lives we have, or for being in the situations we're in. However, when we finally find the courage to relate to ourselves with the unconditional love, kindness, and compassion that we deserve, we can easily see the truth that we all do our best with what we know, and sometimes we don't know what we don't know until we're forced to learn it.

He who learns must suffer
And even in our sleep pain that cannot forget
Falls drop by drop upon the heart
And in our own despite, against our will,
Comes wisdom to us by the awful grace of God.

—AESCHYLUS, ANCIENT GREEK PLAYWRIGHT

Eventually we will all remember that love is the prism through which all of our human needs are met, and through giving ourselves the love we're looking for we can find our way back to the inner peace, health, happiness, and fulfillment that's been alive within us all along. From the very beginning of this universe right through to the beginning of this lifetime, we all take form in the energy of love, which is why, whether we're conscious of it or not, it has always been our destiny to return home to the source of love from which we came, only to realize that we never actually left.

As you can deduce from the title of this book, one of the most important truths I've realized in my own life is that you and I simply were not born to suffer. We did not come into this world to become stuck, numb, unhappy, or unwell. Although many of us have been conditioned to believe that we have to die or be reborn to be free, the truth is that physical death is not the only road to salvation. Our liberation is always available here and now, in this eternal present moment, and all we have to do to welcome it is surrender to the truth, light, and love within us and allow them to fulfill us and heal us completely from the inside out.

When I began to heal and awaken spiritually someone gave me a plaque that said, *"The journey of a thousand miles begins with one step."* The journey back home to our soul after a lifetime of being lost in the material world, in a family, in a relationship, in a job, in an addiction, or in a false image of ourselves is indeed a process. But when we're finally prepared to face our inner suffering head on, we not only find freedom from it quickly, we also prevent further suffering for ourselves as well.

In the end, when we avoid facing what we feel in any given moment or situation, we just prolong our struggle, unhappiness, dis-ease, and insecurity because repressing our uncomfortable emotions only stretches them out over time and blocks us from experiencing our infinite nature. On the other hand, when we choose to face our inner truths directly day in and day out, no matter what, we're always led straight back to the peace, health, happiness, and security we're seeking. Even though this approach to life can seem intense at times, once we fully accept the hurt, anxiety, insecurity, anger, regret, guilt, shame, and fear within us, we can easily move through these emotional storms into the clarity, joy and freedom that are always just beyond the clouds.

As I expressed once before, in my own quest for lasting inner peace, health, happiness, and fulfillment, I have found that underneath my thinking mind and ever-changing emotional state there is an infinite space within me—an underlying and unifying stillness—that is so full of love, joy, and wisdom that no words could ever do justice in communicating this sacred inner truth.

I have no doubt whatsoever that I will "pass over" in this lifetime certain that this space inside of me also exists deep within every single one of us. This place that I'm referring to is so full of unlimited potential, creative intelligence, and vital energy that language does not have words that come close to describing it. I think the most accurate road sign I've ever seen pointing in this direction was when I opened a Chinese fortune cookie and found the following words:

One cloud is enough to eclipse a whole sun.

—Thomas Fuller

In light of how much we suffer over time from a single limiting belief, emotion, unconscious choice, or traumatic experience it is absolutely amazing how true this statement is.

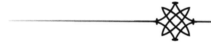

In closing, I'd like to thank you for reading *You Were Not Born to Suffer*. I am eternally grateful that you took the time to love yourself and make our world a healthier and happier place. May you be at peace in your heart, healthy, happy, fulfilled, and free. May you be at home in the source of unconditional love within you and thus love yourself and all life unconditionally. May you be free from your suffering and its causes today and always.

Sincerely with deep love, honor, and gratitude,

Blake D. Bauer

Closing Affirmations

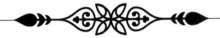

I was not born to suffer.

I deserve the best in all aspects of my life.

I am the love I am seeking.

Today is the first day of the rest of my life.

I remember, and I will never forget.

May I be at peace in my heart, healthy, happy, fulfilled, and free.

May all my loved ones be at peace in their hearts,
healthy, happy, fulfilled, and free.

May all human beings be at peace in their hearts,
healthy, happy, fulfilled, and free.

IN GRATITUDE

I would like to thank the staff at both Balboa Press and Hay House Publishing. I am eternally grateful for your help and guidance in bringing this book to the world.

I would also like to thank Robert Mueller for designing the front and back covers for the 2nd edition of this book. Your amazing work and gift will help this book reach, and thus empower, millions of people all over the world. I am eternally grateful for you sharing your time and magnificent capacities with me. Thank you so very much.

I would also like to thank my beloved mother and father, Abbe and Marshall Bauer, for your support and love over the years. Without you I would not have been able to walk my destined path to the degree that I have, and for this I am eternally grateful. Thank you from the very bottom of my heart.

To Maxine, my beloved partner and best friend, thank you for your love and support. Thank you for unlocking my heart and for reminding me of the infinite source of love that lives within me. Your presence and friendship in my life are blessings indescribable with words.

To my beautiful sister, Cassandra, thank you for your unconditional love and encouragement. You continue to be an amazing friend and inspiration. You mean the world to me, and I am so grateful for your presence in my life. Thank you for choosing me to be your brother. I would not want to live this life without you.

To my late brother, Jason, who I miss so very deeply, thank you for challenging me over the years and for helping me to open my mind to realities I did not know existed. I am eternally grateful that we were brothers in this lifetime, and I look forward to walking in the light with you again when my time and purpose here are complete.

To my late grandmother, Sophie, thank you for your unconditional love, care, and concern. You were an amazing grandmother. Who knows where our entire family would be today had we not had you in our lives?

To the rest of my family, both genetic and soul-based, thank you for being in my life and for teaching me so many lessons about what truly matters.

To all of my ancestors, both biological and spiritual, thank you for paving the way and preparing the soil for me to remember what I had forgotten.

To all of my teachers over the years, thank you for showing up. Without your presence along the way I may have given up on life. I am eternally grateful to each and every one of you.

To all of my beautiful clients past, present, and future, thank you for entrusting me with the honor of witnessing and supporting you in your healing and awakening. I am eternally grateful. You humble me and you make my life largely worth living. From the bottom of my heart, thank you.

Last but not least, to you the reader, thank you for sharing your journey with me, and thank you for allowing me to share my journey with you. I am honored.

ABOUT THE AUTHOR

Blake D. Bauer is an internationally recognized author, spiritual teacher, and alternative medicine practitioner. His pioneering work centers on loving yourself unconditionally as the key to healing yourself, fulfilling your life's purpose, and realizing your greatest potential both personally and professionally. Based on his training with spiritual teachers, healers, and masters from all over the world, Blake practices and teaches various forms of meditation, qi gong, qi gong energy medicine, and dao yin (a health and longevity yoga). Blake's formal education also includes traditional Chinese medicine, five-element Chinese medicine, nutritional medicine, herbal healing, psychology, past life 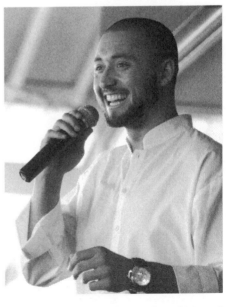 regression therapy-hypnosis, and various other forms of traditional healing and alternative medicine. Bringing together the most effective spiritual practices and holistic approaches to health and wellbeing, Blake's work and teachings have successfully guided thousands of people internationally toward greater psychological, emotional, physical, financial, and spiritual freedom.

For more information on Blake Bauer and his work, please visit: www.unconditional-selflove.com.

BLAKE BAUER TEACHINGS

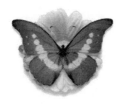

Wisdom From The Heart – Freedom For The Soul™

Guidance and Healing for Total Life Transformation

Self-Awareness—Self-Love—Self-Healing—
Self-Mastery—Self-Realization

Private Healing and Counseling
Personal and Professional Success Coaching
Evolutionary Energetic Medicine™
Past Life Regression Therapy, Healing, and Hypnosis
Meditation
Qi Gong—Therapeutic Healing Exercises
Workshops
Seminars
Retreats
Professional Trainings
Evolutionary Business Coaching and Consulting
Personal Development

please visit:

www.unconditional-selflove.com

NOTES

NOTES

NOTES

NOTES

Made in the USA
Lexington, KY
09 July 2014